HOW TO DIAGN
LIKE A DOCTOR
ON YOUR FIRST DAY
IN MEDICAL SCHOOL

Frank J. Slaby, Ph.D.

Professor

Department of Anatomy & Regenerative Biology

George Washington University School of Medicine

Washington, D.C.

ISBN-10 1484914937
ISBN-13 978-1484914939

Copyright 2013 by FJS Ventures, LLC

This book is a publication of FJS Ventures, LLC, and is protected by copyright. All rights reserved. Except as permitted under the Copyright Act of 1976, no part of this publication may be reproduced or distributed in any form or by any means or stored in a database or retrieval system, without the prior written permission of the author.

DEDICATION

The author dedicates this book to his wife, Susan K. McCune, M.D., and our son, Christopher. Their support and assistance lightened and speeded the effort.

DISCLAIMER

The author has attempted to provide the most accurate information regarding the cognitive steps by which experienced physicians efficiently and effectively diagnose disease and injury and how medical students can learn the basic medical sciences in medical school in relation to the clinical findings of patients. However, the author and the publisher are not responsible for errors or omissions and in no way should the information provided in this book be applied to diagnose or treat patients or substitute for modern clinical training. The author and publisher make no warranty, expressed or implied, with respect to the accuracy or application of the information contained in this book in the diagnosis and treatment of patients.

TABLE OF CONTENTS

HOW TO DIAGNOSE LIKE A DOCTOR
ON YOUR FIRST DAY IN MEDICAL SCHOOL

Chapter 1

DATA ACQUISITION

This book is written to be a fast read for you, a first-year medical student. Hopefully, you are reading this book just before you begin your first year of medical school or are in the midst of your first semester in medical school, as you need to know up front that one of the most critical evaluations of your performance in medical school will be the assessment of your diagnostic reasoning skills during your clinical clerkships. This is a major component of how clinical instructors really evaluate your knowledge fund and analytical skills, because "diagnosis is at the core of medical practice."[1-1] The strength of your diagnostic reasoning or lack thereof provides testimony of your ability to recall basic medical science knowledge and apply it to the analysis of a patient's condition.

The central theme of this book is that there is a critical fault in the curriculum of almost all medical schools in the United States today, namely, that medical students are not provided the opportunity to learn the basic medical sciences, such as gross anatomy, microscopic anatomy, biochemistry, physiology, immunology, and neurobiology, in relation to the clinical findings of patients, and that this fault severely restricts the development of diagnostic reasoning skills in medical school. The principal argument of this book is that you, a first-year medical student, can independently and at least partly remedy this fault by adopting a few simple study habits all throughout your medical school years. These study habits are based upon our current understanding of some of the principal practices that experienced physicians employ to efficiently and accurately diagnose illness and injury. The principal thesis of this book is thus that, if you understand the nature of these diagnostic practices before you begin medical school and start employing them upon beginning medical school, they will help you learn the basic medical sciences in relation to the clinical findings of patients and noticeably advance the development of your diagnostic reasoning skills in medical school.

So that you may understand the rationale for the structure of your school's curriculum, we begin here in Chapter 1 with a discussion of the origin of the basic four-year curriculum that is offered in almost all medical schools in the United States today. Our first medical school was founded in 1765 in association with both the College of Philadelphia (the predecessor of the University of Pennsylvania) and the Pennsylvania Hospital in Philadelphia. Its purpose was to provide a modicum of instruction that supplemented the traditional method of medical education: apprenticeship. A medical education was gained throughout the 18th Century and even most of the 19th Century primarily through several years of apprenticeship to an experienced physician. The physician served as a preceptor who provided almost all the practical experience and training necessary to become a doctor of medicine.

In 1852, the newly constituted American Medical Association (the AMA) proposed national educational standards for a degree in medicine. The standards included completion of first a course of study in subjects such as anatomy, medicine, surgery, and chemistry in a medical school to be followed by 2 years apprenticeship to a qualified physician. By 1900, however, the establishment of new medical schools had become so proliferate and their curricular standards so irregular that the AMA's Council on Medical Education requested the Carnegie Foundation to support a thorough study of the state of medical education throughout the United States and Canada. As a result, in 1908, the Carnegie Foundation commissioned Abraham Flexner, a non-physician, progressive educator, to survey all 155 medical schools in the United States and Canada and prepare a report with recommendations for improvement and standardization of medical education.

Flexner surveyed all 155 medical schools and found that they varied in quality from excellent to scandalous. There was no standardization of the course of study among the medical schools nor any rigorous qualifications required of medical school instructors. Confounding this chaotic state of medical education was the relatively primitive state of medical knowledge and patient examination techniques at that time. The only basic medical sciences that were even moderately well developed by today's standards were the anatomical sciences, such as gross anatomy and histology. The concept that physical examination of a patient should be the keystone of diagnosis had not gained general acceptance until the 1850's.[1-2] The germ theory of disease had not begun to influence the practice of medicine until the 1870's. Use of the binaural stethoscope in the physical examination of patients did not become common until the 1890's.[1-3] Radiology was in its infancy, as recognition that X-rays could be used to image internal anatomy did not occur until 1895.[1-4] Electrocardiography had only been recently discovered in 1901. Although it was known that inherited traits are transmitted via discrete units in cells, the chemical nature of the discrete units, genes, would not become firmly established until the 1940's.

Flexner reported his findings in 1910, and they were a bombshell. He described the outlandishly corrupt practices at the medical schools that operated as diploma mills; these schools basically required nothing more than full payment of the tuition for issuance of an M.D. degree. He also lauded the attributes and professional dedication of the paragon institution of medical education: the Johns Hopkins University School of Medicine. The most profound contribution of his report, though, was his identification of a straightforward curricular solution to the medical education demands of the period. His solution stemmed from his prescient appreciation that medical practice would increasingly become based upon scientific principles and technological developments. He thus proposed that medical school should be a 4-year program of study that is divided into an initial 2-year period dedicated to the learning of the basic medical sciences to be followed by a 2-year period of clinical exposure. Here are his exact words:

> "For purposes of convenience, the medical curriculum may be divided into two parts, according as the work is carried on mainly in laboratories or mainly in the hospital; but the distinction is superficial, for the hospital is itself in the fullest sense a laboratory. In general, the four-year curriculum falls into two fairly equal sections: the first two years are devoted mainly to laboratory sciences,-anatomy, physiology, pharmacology, pathology; the last two to clinical work in medicine, surgery, and obstetrics. The former are concerned with the study of normal and abnormal phenomena as such; the latter are busy with their practical treatment as manifested in disease."[1-5]

Flexner described the basic medical sciences as laboratory sciences because he believed that the laboratory exercises associated with each basic medical science course provided the means by which medical students learned the nature of scientific investigation and appreciated the scientific basis of medical knowledge. He also recommended that all medical schools be associated with a university in order to ensure high academic standards. The standards for excellence in medical education established by Flexner account for the fact that, a century later, the first 18 to 24 months of the curriculum in almost all United States medical schools are dedicated to the teaching of the basic medical sciences by instructors with Ph.D. degrees in these fields.

Instruction by physicians does not become dominant in medical schools today until medical students begin their clinical clerkships during the latter half of their second year or the beginning of the third year. At this juncture, most medical students know how to take a patient's present, past, and family medical history and how to perform a basic physical exam. However, they have little, if any, experience examining real patients in an office or hospital setting and virtually no instruction in how to organize their diagnostic reasoning. As they encounter real patients in their clinical clerkships, clinical instructors challenge the medical students directly to explain how they are thinking about each patient's condition, given the patient's history and physical examination and, for some patients, radiological findings and lab test results. In effect, this becomes the time in medical school that most medical students identify as the beginning of the development of their diagnostic reasoning skills.

However, you should understand that your diagnostic reasoning skills really begin when you receive your first sessions on how to take a patient's present, past, and family medical history and perform a basic physical exam. These sessions are typically dispersed throughout the first 18 to 24 months of the curriculum. Your competency in these skills determines the accuracy and thoroughness of the information you can acquire about a patient's health. From a practical point of view, what you ultimately think about a patient's health is strictly dependent upon what you know factually about a patient's health, and this factual information begins with the data acquired during the history and physical exam.

The first 18 to 24 months of the curriculum in most medical schools today are thus focused on two broad learning objectives: (1) an ability to recall basic medical science knowledge and (2) an ability to acquire from the history, physical exam, and medical records of a patient all appropriate data relevant to the patient's medical problems. The level of competency that you attain in the performance of these two abilities prior to beginning your clinical clerkships is the cognitive foundation upon which you develop higher-order medical diagnostic reasoning skills. Other cognitive skills associated with diagnostic reasoning are typically not identified as major learning objectives during the first 18 to 24 months of the curriculum in most medical schools today.

RREFERENCES

1-1. Charlin B, Tardif J, and H Boshuizen. Scripts and Medical Knowledge: Theory and Applications for Clinical Reasoning Instruction and Research. Academic Medicine (2000) 75:182-190. p. 183.

1-2. Reiser, SJ. Medicine and the Reign of Technology (1978) Cambridge University Press. p. 38.

1-3. Reiser, SJ. Medicine and the Reign of Technology (1978) Cambridge University Press. p. 43.

1-4. Reiser, SJ. Technological Medicine: The Changing World of Doctors and Patients (2009) Cambridge University Press. p. 15.

1-5. Flexner, A. Medical Education in the United States and Canada: A Report to the Carnegie Foundation for the Advancement of Teaching. (1910) p. 57.

Chapter 2

HYPOTHETICAL-DEDUCTIVE REASONING

As noted on page 9, Abraham Flexner based his proposal for medical school curricular reform on his belief that medical practice in the 20th Century would be guided increasingly by scientific knowledge. Hypothetical-deductive reasoning is one of the most basic analytical approaches by which scientific knowledge is acquired. Hypothetical-deductive reasoning in scientific research employs a three-step process:

(1) The investigator identifies a hypothesis to be tested,

(2) The investigator deduces a prediction of the hypothesis, and then

(3) The investigator conducts an experiment whose results either support or controvert the prediction.

Scientific knowledge is based on scientific theories, which, in turn, are generated mainly by hypothetical-deductive reasoning. Scientific theories are advanced when scientists infer predictions of the theories and then confirm by experimental studies the validity of the predictions. A scientific theory becomes overturned or modified if an experimental study controverts one of its inferred predictions.

When medical students are asked in their clinical clerkships to generate likely diagnoses on real patients, they are advised to adopt hypothetical-deductive reasoning. To employ hypothetical-deductive reasoning when examining a real patient, a medical student must be able first to recall basic medical science knowledge, such as knowledge of anatomy, biochemistry, genetics, physiology, immunology, microbiology, pathophysiology, and pharmacology. A medical student must then be able to apply the basic medical science knowledge to account for the pathophysiological mechanisms that have generated the signs, symptoms, and abnormal physical exam findings of the patient's ill health [symptoms are problems that the patient self-identifies; signs are problems that you, as the examiner, identify during the history and physical exam]. This dependency of hypothetical-deductive reasoning on recall and application of basic medical science knowledge accounts for the 18 to 24-month delay in initiating diagnostic reasoning development in most medical schools today.

Hypothetical-deductive reasoning is the most basic diagnostic reasoning strategy that an examiner (be it a medical student, resident, or experienced physician) can employ. As Flexner foresaw, it is an analytical approach that draws upon scientific knowledge. Hypothetical-deductive reasoning is always used to select the tests that either support or controvert a proposed diagnosis.

To appreciate how a medical student might employ hypothetical-deductive reasoning to diagnose a patient's problem, consider the following fictional case: The patient is a 20 year-old male who presents with one chief complaint: a sore left wrist. The medical student learns from the history that the patient's left wrist began hurting after the patient fell down on his outstretched left hand while playing basketball. The patient describes the pain as a deep, dull ache in the wrist that intensifies with hand movements. The patient does not report any abnormal sensations, such as pain or numbness, in the palm of the hand, the dorsum of the hand (that is, the back of the hand), the thumb, or the fingers. Physical examination finds that the patient can perform all movements of the hand at the left wrist, but some movements evoke increased pain. The patient can perform all thumb and finger movements in the left hand without any pain or weakness. On the basis of this information, the medical student concludes that whatever the nature of the patient's injury, it does not appear to have resulted in any sensory (that is, nerve-related) or motor (that is, muscle-related) deficits in the left hand. The medical student recalls that the only wrist injuries discussed in either the gross anatomy course or the physical exam sessions were fractures and dislocations of the small bones in the wrist; these bones are called the carpals. The medical student recalls that the most commonly fractured carpal is the scaphoid, and the most commonly dislocated carpal is the lunate. The medical student also recalls that a common mechanism by which the scaphoid is fractured or the lunate dislocated is by a fall on an outstretched hand (a Fall On an OutStretched Hand is abbreviated in clinical notes as a FOOSH).

Based on the patient's history and physical exam and the medical student's recall of relevant gross anatomy knowledge, the student hypothesizes that the patient may have a fractured scaphoid or a dislocated lunate. The student recalls from physical examination training that there is a physical examination test, which, if positive, is almost pathognomonic for a fractured scaphoid [the word 'pathognomonic' refers to a feature or test result which is specifically distinctive of a disease or injury]. In this physical exam test, an examiner's index finger is pressed onto a hollowed-out area on the side of the patient's wrist near the base of the thumb; this hollowed-out area is called the anatomical snuffbox. If this test is performed on a patient with a history suggesting a fractured scaphoid, and the pressure on the anatomical snuffbox elicits increased pain in the wrist, then it is highly likely that the patient has a fractured scaphoid. The student recalls from the gross anatomy course that a diagnosis of a dislocated lunate is best tested by examination of radiographs of the patient's injured wrist. In this case, because the physical exam test for a fractured scaphoid can be readily performed in the examination room, the student performs the test and finds that it evokes increased pain in the patient's left wrist, thus supporting the diagnosis of a fractured scaphoid.

This case illustrates the validity of hypothetical-deductive reasoning as the analytical basis of diagnostic reasoning. The student combined the knowledge learned from the patient's history and physical exam with the knowledge learned from gross anatomy studies and physical examination training to generate two hypotheses: the patient has either a fractured scaphoid or a dislocated lunate in his left wrist. The student then deduced that if the patient has a fractured scaphoid, pressure applied to the anatomical snuffbox of the patient's left wrist should elicit increased pain. The positive test result supported the diagnosis of a fractured scaphoid. It should be noted, however, that, if this were a real patient, a number of radiographs of the patient's left wrist would be examined to confirm this tentative diagnosis. Scaphoid fractures are frequently difficult to discern 1 to 2 days after the injury because many scaphoid fractures are hairline, undisplaced fractures. In cases in which a scaphoid fracture is strongly suspected but not radiographically confirmed, the wrist is immobilized in a plaster cast (to provide the appropriate conditions for union of the proximal and distal fragments), and radiographic evaluation is repeated 7 to 10 days later. The subsequent bone resorption that occurs at the fracture site renders the site more apparent in the latter set of radiographs.

This fractured scaphoid case also illustrates another hallmark feature of diagnostic reasoning: as an examiner acquires information during the history and physical exam, the examiner begins positing possible diagnoses during the history and physical exam. This is as true of medical students as it is of residents and experienced physicians. The generation of possible diagnoses during the history and physical exam may occur at a subconscious level.

When you get to the end of this book and learn about the most elaborate diagnostic reasoning strategies that experienced physicians employ while examining patients, you will realize that their diagnostic reasoning strategies are all built upon the foundation of hypothetical-deductive reasoning. This is because although their diagnostic reasoning strategies may be very elaborate, in the end, they generate 1, 2, or more hypotheses, which then have to be challenged by appropriate tests.

In general, however, employing just hypothetical-deductive reasoning to diagnose a patient's problems is not an effective strategy. This is because many patients present with one or more problems whose genesis is not as apparent as in the fractured scaphoid case. This is especially true of patients with chronic diseases or hospitalized patients. Consequently, when medical students begin examining real patients in their clinical clerkships, they find diagnosis to be a difficult and frustrating task. As students attempt to generate a hypothetical pathophysiological mechanism or injury that has led to a patient's ill health, they commonly find that what they learn from a patient's history and physical exam as well as radiological findings and lab test results does not readily trigger recall of related basic medical science knowledge. Their recall of basic medical science knowledge is poor because it was presented and learned during the first 18 to 24 months of medical school in relation to the structure of the students' basic medical science courses instead of in relation to the clinical findings of patients.[2-1] Because the cues for recall are different, recall tends to be slow, incomplete, and occasionally irrelevant. As Denson has explained:

> "Clinical expertise is linked to having well-organized knowledge. As students acquire knowledge, they organize it into schemes. In the typical "2+2" medical curriculum (2 years of basic science followed by 2 years of clinical rotations), students acquire information in each of a number of disciplines over the first 2 years. In contrast, as students travel from one clinical clerkship to the next, they encounter patients with specialty-specific complaints. The first of these realities imposes a discipline-based organizing scheme, whereas the second imparts a complaint-based scheme. In such curricula, it is largely left to the student to form the connections that integrate discipline-based knowledge with patient complaint/disease-focused information."[2-2]

This then is the basic conundrum of medical education today: Whereas basic medical science knowledge is the basis of the foundation upon which a medical student develops a diagnostic reasoning process, basic medical science knowledge cannot be efficiently and effectively accessed and utilized when examining patients if it is not learned in relation to the clinical findings of patients. It is noteworthy that Flexner appreciated a hundred years ago that the basic medical sciences should be learned in medical school in relation to their application to medical care. Immediately after proposing that a 4-year medical school curriculum should be evenly divided between an initial 2-year period of basic medical science instruction and a concluding 2-year period of clinical exposure, he asks:

"How far the earlier years [the first 2 years] should be at all conscious of the latter [the last 2 years] is a mooted question. Anatomy and physiology are ultimately biological sciences. Do the professional purposes of the medical school modify the strict biological point of view? Should the teaching of anatomy and physiology be affected by the fact that these subjects are parts of a medical curriculum? Or ought they be presented exactly as they would be presented to students of biology not intending to be physicians? A layman hesitates to offer an opinion where the doctors disagree, but the purely pedagogical standpoint may assist a determination of the issue."[2-3]

As he then considers the issue, he observes that

"These considerations, however, still omit one highly important fact: medical education is a technical or professional discipline; it calls for the possession of certain portions of many sciences arranged and organized with a distinct practical purpose in view. That's what makes it a 'profession.' Its point of view is not that of any one of the sciences as such. It is difficult to see how separate acquisitions in several fields can be organically combined, can be brought to play upon each other, in the realization of a controlling purpose, unless this purpose is consciously present in the selection and manipulation of the material."[2-4]

On the next page he finally draws his conclusion:

"Undergraduate instruction [that is, instruction in the basic medical sciences] will be throughout explicitly conscious of its professional end and aim. In no other way can all the sciences belonging to the medical curriculum be thoroughly kneaded. An active apperceptive relation must by established and maintained between laboratory and clinical experience. Such a relation cannot be one-sided; it will not spontaneously set itself up in the last two years if it is deliberately suppressed in the first two. There is no cement like interest, no stimulus like the hint of a coming practical application."[2-5]

Flexner notes in his 1910 report that medical schools may have to resort to securing non-physicians for basic medical science instruction: "There is no question that these posts (that is, the posts for teaching the basic medical sciences) cannot be satisfactorily filled by active physicians."[2-6] And this is exactly what occurred as the 20th Century unfolded: Men and women with doctoral degrees in the basic medical sciences were increasingly recruited to teach the basic medical science courses in medical school. As the pace of biomedical research progressively increased, especially following the availability of radioactive chemicals for biomedical research and the development of the electron microscope after World War II, it became increasingly difficult for practicing physicians to keep pace with the most recent research discoveries in the basic medical sciences. This limitation led to the active recruitment of research-active Ph.D.s in the basic medical sciences to teach these subjects in medical school. Consequently, instruction in the basic medical science courses became increasingly framed in terms of biomedical research theory and progressively less framed in terms of the clinical findings of patients.

Three developments during the past 50 years have shed light on the critical importance of medical students learning the basic medical sciences in terms of the clinical findings of patients. The first is the development of an adult learning theory called andragogy by the American educator Malcolm Knowles. "Andragogy makes the following assumptions about the design of adult learning: (1) Adults need to know why they need to learn something, (2) Adults need to learn experientially, (3) Adults approach learning as problem-solving, and (4) Adults learn best when the topic is of immediate value. In practical terms, andragogy means that instruction for adults needs to focus more on the process and less on the content being taught."[2-7] Knowles' andragogy theory led to the phrase 'an instructor for adults needs to be a guide by the side instead of a sage on the stage.' In formulating his theory of adult learning, Knowles recognized that adult learners are both self-motivated and self-directed. As such, they know where to find content, be it a book, a website, or an expert in the field of interest. Adult learners want their instructors to be experienced in providing guidance on how to apply newly-gained knowledge to solve real-life problems, for it is through this experience that adult learners develop the ability to apply their knowledge. "Adult learning theory holds that people learn new knowledge and skills most effectively when they are presented in the context of application of new knowledge to real-life situations."[2-8] Andragogy applies, in particular, to medical students, as they are young adult learners who seek primarily to learn how to diagnose and treat illness and injury. Their interest is focused, for example, not on anatomical or physiological knowledge by itself, but rather on how that knowledge is employed to diagnose and treat illness and injury. To paraphrase Flexner's words, a medical education's 'point of view is not that of any one of the sciences as such.'

The second development has been the startling, ever-accelerating pace at which medical knowledge has been increasing.

> "It is estimated that the doubling time of medical knowledge in 1950 was 50 years; in 1980, 7 years; and in 2010, 3.5 years. In 2020 it is projected to be 0.2 years-just 73 days. Students who began medical school in the autumn of 2010 will experience approximately 3 doublings in knowledge by the time they complete the minimum length of training (7 years) needed to practice medicine. Students who graduate in 2020 will experience 4 doublings in knowledge. What was learned in the first 3 years of medical school will be just 6% of what is known at the end of the decade from 2010 to 2020. Knowledge is expanding faster than our ability to assimilate and apply it effectively; and this is as true in education and patient care as it is in research. Clearly, simply adding more material and/or time to the curriculum will not be an effective coping strategy-fundamental change has become an imperative."[2-9]

Near the beginning of the 20th Century it was reasonable for Flexner to contend not only that a medical student could learn much, if not most, of the basic medical sciences during the first two years of medical school but also that acquisition of such knowledge was a necessary requirement of a proper medical education. It is obvious now near the beginning of the 21st Century that requiring students to learn each basic medical science in the context of a discipline-based course not only is not pedagogically sound but also is a practical impossibility. The challenge for medical educators today is to define and redefine every few years the relatively minute body of basic medical scientific knowledge that is a necessary requirement of a proper medical education.

The third development is the growing consensus among investigators of diagnostic reasoning that the diagnostic skills of a medical examiner, be it a medical student, a resident, or an experienced physician, can be understood in terms of contemporary theories in cognitive psychology. "Cognitive psychologists generally assume that the knowledge people acquire about the world is organized or packaged into cognitive models. These are mental representations at some level of abstraction of objects or events encountered in, or learned about, the outer world."[2-10] Investigations of experienced physicians indicate that, when operating in their field of diagnostic expertise, they tend to employ certain well-defined cognitive steps to arrive at a diagnosis of a patient's illness or injury. Like medical students examining their first patients in clinical clerkships, their first step is to acquire from the history, physical exam, lab tests, and medical records of a patient all appropriate data relevant to the patient's medical problems. However, even as experienced physicians are in the midst of examining their patients, they begin drawing from their memory knowledge structures called illness scripts.[2-11] Each illness script is regarded as a potential diagnosis because it designates a disease or injury whose manifestations closely resemble those of the patient being examined. The illness script whose characteristics most closely match those of the patient being examined is commonly chosen as the most likely diagnosis. Illness scripts are believed to be the cognitive structures that account for the efficiency by which experienced physicians arrive at accurate diagnoses. Illness scripts are personal knowledge structures that each physician develops and continuously refines through the experience of examining first hundreds and then thousands of patients.

The ability to effectively and accurately recall basic medical science knowledge when examining patients is key to both diagnostic efficiency and diagnostic accuracy. The recognition that experienced physicians employ illness scripts to efficiently and accurately diagnose their patients implies that diagnostic reasoning skills are acquired through the development of cognitive models that become progressively more elaborate as medical students proceed through medical school, residency, and the first years of clinical practice.[2-12] The principal argument of this book is that the development and refinement of these cognitive models should be a major learning objective throughout all four years of medical school. To do this, the learning of the basic medical sciences in relation to the clinical findings of patients should begin in the first semester of medical school. This is exactly what Flexner proposed and adult learning theory suggests is the optimal learning strategy for medical students throughout the four years of medical school. The following three chapters address what you need to do to structure your basic medical science knowledge in relation to the clinical findings of patients.

REFERENCES

2-1. Bowen, JL. Educational Strategies to Promote Clinical Diagnostic Reasoning. New England Journal of Medicine (2006) 355:2217-2225 p. 2217.

2-2. Densen P. Challenges and Opportunities Facing Medical Education. Transactions of the American Clinical and Climatological Association. (2011) 122:48-58. p. 51.

2-3. Flexner, A. Medical Education in the United States and Canada: A Report to the Carnegie Foundation for the Advancement of Teaching. (1910) p. 57.

2-4. Flexner, A. Medical Education in the United States and Canada: A Report to the Carnegie Foundation for the Advancement of Teaching. (1910) p. 58.

2-5. Flexner, A. Medical Education in the United States and Canada: A Report to the Carnegie Foundation for the Advancement of Teaching. (1910) p. 59.

2-6. Flexner, A. Medical Education in the United States and Canada: A Report to the Carnegie Foundation for the Advancement of Teaching. (1910) p. 72.

2-7. http://www.instructionaldesign.org/theories/andragogy.html

2-8. Kassirer, JP. Teaching Clinical Reasoning: Case-Based and Coached. Academic Medicine (2010) 85:1118-1124 pp. 1118 and 1119.

2-9. Densen P. Challenges and Opportunities Facing Medical Education. Transactions of the American Clinical and Climatological Association. (2011) 122:48-58. pp. 50 & 51.

2-10. Schmidt HG, Norman GR, and HPA Boshuizen. A Cognitive Perspective on Medical Expertise: Theory and Implications. Academic Medicine (1990) 65:611-621 p. 613.

2-11. Feltovich PJ and HS Barrows. Issues of Generality in Medical Problem Solving. In: Schmidt HG and ML DeVolder eds. Tutorials in Problem-Based Learning. Assen/Maastricht: Van Gorcum (1984) pp. 128–142.

2-12. Schmidt HG, Norman GR, and HPA Boshuizen. A Cognitive Perspective on Medical Expertise: Theory and Implications. Academic Medicine (1990) 65:611-621.

Chapter 3

SEMANTIC QUALIFIERS AND PROBLEM REPRESENTATIONS

Semantics is the field of linguistics that focuses on the study of meaning in language. The expression semantic qualifiers, when discussed in reference to the practice of medicine, refer to words heavily laden with diagnostic meaning. For example, if you are examining a patient with a major complaint of pain somewhere in the body, one of the most important questions you should ask about the pain is whether it began very recently or has been present for some time. Pain that began within the last few days is described as acute pain. In contrast, pain which has been present, either continuously or intermittently, for weeks or even months is described as chronic pain. In medical diagnostic reasoning, the pair of terms acute & chronic is referred to as a pair of semantic qualifiers. Observe that semantic qualifiers are pairs of terms that bear opposite meanings. This is the critical characteristic of semantic qualifiers.[3-1] The oppositional meanings of a pair of semantic qualifiers are the basis of the potency of their diagnostic meaning. This is because whereas one member of a pair of semantic qualifiers tends to draw your attention to a particular class of likely diagnoses, the other member tends to draw your attention to a different class of likely diagnoses.

When you examine a patient, you want to establish as many semantic qualifiers of the patient's condition as possible. This rule applies to each of the patient's signs and symptoms. The more semantic qualifiers that you can gather about a patient's symptom or sign, the greater are their aggregate diagnostic value. For example, there are many other semantic qualifiers that you should inquire about when examining a patient with pain. Is the pain sharp, like a small cut on a finger, or a dull ache? Is the pain distinctly localized or diffuse? Is the pain intense or mild? Is the pain constant or intermittent? Is there a movement that intensifies or minimizes the pain? Is there a body position that intensifies or minimizes the pain? If there a movement or body position that changes the location of the pain? As you compile as many semantic qualifiers of a patient's pain as you can, you are, in effect, progressively whittling down the most likely diagnoses to just those which are suggested by the specific set of semantic qualifiers that characterize the patient's pain.

The identification of the semantic qualifiers of a patient's signs and symptoms represents the first cognitive step of diagnostic reasoning by an experienced physician. This first cognitive step is critical because the semantic qualifiers form the basic elements of the second cognitive step of diagnostic reasoning: the construction of a problem representation of the patient's condition (Fig. 3-1).[3-2] Experienced physicians recognize that semantic qualifiers are abbreviated descriptors of a patient's signs and symptoms. Consequently, when an experienced physician completes an examination of a patient, the physician uses the semantic qualifiers of the patient's condition to construct a succinct description of the patient called a problem representation.[3-3] The problem representation typically consists of 1 or 2 sentences that summarize the most diagnostically relevant features of the patient's condition. A well-constructed problem representation is typically liberally populated with semantic qualifiers.

STEP 1:   Identify the semantic qualifiers of
                           the patient's signs and symptoms

                                      ↓

STEP 2:   Construct the patient's problem representation:
                    A 1 or 2 sentence description of the patient's condition
                    that is liberally populated with the semantic qualifiers
                           of the patient's signs and symptoms

              Fig 3-1: The first two cognitive steps of diagnostic reasoning
                           by an experienced physician.

Experienced physicians use problem representations rich in semantic qualifiers as a critical cognitive step in diagnostic reasoning. When you begin examining patients during your clinical clerkships, the most revealing indicator of your diagnostic reasoning will be the quality of your problem representations. At that time, your clinical instructors will expect that you have some degree of proficiency with really only one cognitive step of diagnostic reasoning: data acquisition. They can evaluate your ability to take an appropriate history and competently perform a basic physical exam by asking you to present the results of your examination of a patient whose medical condition has already been assessed by a physician. If you are next asked to describe your thoughts about the patient, they expect that you will begin attempting to use hypothetical-deductive reasoning to account for the patient's condition. However, that is not what an experienced physician would do. An experienced physician recognizes that after gathering all the data about a patient, the next cognitive step of diagnostic reasoning is to construct a succinct, objective problem representation heavily populated with semantic qualifiers. This is because the problem representation presents in abbreviated terms all of the patient's medical problems that define the patient's condition. It is this abbreviated, objective definition of the patient's condition that is the appropriate starting point in an experienced physician's mind to begin the search for the most likely diagnoses.

There is a very important reason why experienced physicians place so much emphasis on the construction of a well-crafted problem representation of a patient. It retrieves from the experienced physician's memory the illness scripts with similar problem representations. For an experienced physician, problem representations serve as the diagnostic tags of illness scripts. In the mind of an experienced physician, each illness script is the cognitive structure in which is embedded not only the pathophysiology of a disease or injury but also the conditions that predispose a person to a disease or injury. Recognize that this is another argument why you should learn the basic medical sciences in medical school in terms of the clinical findings of patients. It is because as you gain experience in abbreviating and condensing the clinical findings of a patient into a problem representation rich in semantic qualifiers, you will use the problem representation to help you recall the illness script that best fits the problem representation, which, in turn, will aid your recall of the predisposing factors and pathophysiology. Consequently, you want to start medical school by learning the basic medical sciences in terms of the cues that you will use to recall this knowledge as you proceed through medical school, residency, and medical practice.

In order to appreciate how semantic qualifiers facilitate the construction of a succinct problem representation of a patient's condition, consider the following fictional case: A 22 year-old male enters the emergency room at 10 PM complaining of abdominal pain. The following is a transcript of the history taken by the attending second-year resident and a summary of the physical exam findings:

What has brought you to the ER tonight?

- A bad pain in my belly.

Where does it hurt?

- Over here (the patient circles his right hand around the region of his abdomen just above the umbilicus).

When did the pain start?

- Around 7 this morning, right after I got up.

How would you describe the pain?

- It's like a deep ache that never goes away.

Has the nature of the pain or its location changed since this morning?

- No, not really.

Have you ever had a pain like this before?

- Yes, when I had the stomach flu or somethin' like it, but it's never been as constant as this time.

Is there anything that makes the pain worse?

- No.

Is there anything that relieves the pain?

- No.

Is there anything else that is also bothering you, or that you think may be associated with your belly pain?

- I don't know. I haven't felt like eating since this morning, and, on and off, I have felt nauseous. But I haven't vomited anything.

Do you know any people around you, such as members of your family or friends, who have also recently suffered from belly pain?

- No.

Have you traveled out of the area or taken a vacation recently?

- No.

Are you taking any medications?

- No.

Physical Exam Findings: Vital signs are normal except for a temperature of 101.5°F. System exams are normal except for tenderness to deep palpation in the right lower quadrant (RLQ) of the abdomen [the RLQ of the abdomen is the quarter of the abdomen below the umbilicus and to the right of the midline of the body].

Before turning the page, try to write 1 or 2 sentences with semantic qualifiers that succinctly describe the patient's condition.

The following statement is an appropriate problem representation of the patient: The patient is a 22 year-old, febrile, anorexic male with diffuse, dull periumbilical pain of 15 hours duration and right lower quadrant (RLQ) tenderness upon deep palpation. [Periumbilical pain is pain around the umbilicus.]

Observe first that a problem presentation should always specify the age and sex of the patient. Next, observe that the problem presentation in this case characterizes the patient's condition by his four abnormal signs and symptoms: (1) the patient has moderately intense abdominal pain (it is of sufficient intensity to have compelled the patient to visit the ER), (2) the patient is anorexic (the pain has discouraged the patient from eating), (3) the patient is febrile (he has a low grade fever), and (4) the patient has abdominal tenderness when the examiner's hands are pressed deeply into the RLQ of the patient's abdomen. Finally, observe that the abdominal pain is characterized by five semantic qualifiers: (1) it is moderately intense, (2) it is dull, like a stomach ache, (2) it is experienced over a relatively wide area in the abdomen, as opposed to a specific point, (3) the center of the diffuse, dull painful area is just above the umbilicus, and (4) the pain has been unrelenting during the past 15 hours.

A senior level medical student would recognize that the patient is most likely suffering from an acute appendicitis (that is, acute inflammation of the appendix). Before discussing how a senior-level medical student would arrive at this diagnosis and the critical role that a problem representation plays in diagnostic reasoning, let's first discuss the appendix and the nature of acute appendicitis.

The drawing on the following page shows an anterior, or frontal, view of the large intestine as it lies in the abdomen (Fig. 3-1). The appendix is a worm-like appendage of the large intestine located at the lower end of the right side of the large intestine. Acute appendicitis is the condition in which the appendix becomes inflamed and swollen. Acute appendicitis is caused by blockage of the lumen, or interior, of the appendix; there are a number of conditions which can cause blockage. If the blockage persists, the appendix begins to swell because of an increase of fluid within the interior of the appendix. At the same time, the proliferation of intestinal bacteria within the interior of the appendix leads to inflammation of the appendix, that is, acute appendicitis. Inflammation is the process by which the body recruits cells and factors from the blood to control and repair tissues damaged by disease or injury. Appendectomy (surgical removal of the appendix) is the only curative treatment of appendicitis.

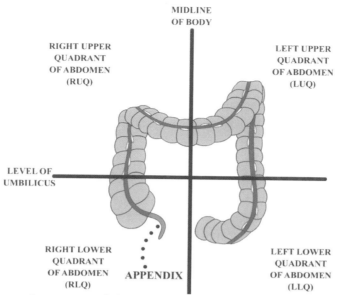

MIDLINE OF BODY

RIGHT UPPER QUADRANT OF ABDOMEN (RUQ)

LEFT UPPER QUADRANT OF ABDOMEN (LUQ)

LEVEL OF UMBILICUS

RIGHT LOWER QUADRANT OF ABDOMEN (RLQ)

APPENDIX

LEFT LOWER QUADRANT OF ABDOMEN (LLQ)

Fig. 3-1: Anterior view of the appendix in the RLQ of the abdomen.

At this point, you may be asking yourself "why is diffuse periumbilical pain the first indication of acute appendicitis if the appendix is in the right lower quadrant of the abdomen?" Although the anatomical basis of this early symptom is not completely understood, the following is the generally accepted explanation: The appendix is innervated by sensory nerve fibers (called visceral sensory nerve fibers) that enter the spinal cord at primarily the segment of the spinal cord from which the 10th thoracic spinal nerves arise; this spinal cord segment is called the T10 segment. The horizontal band of skin in the anterior abdominal wall (the anterior abdominal wall is the wall of skin and muscles which covers the front of the abdomen) that lies at the level of the umbilicus is innervated by sensory nerve fibers (called somatic sensory nerve fibers) that also enter the spinal cord at primarily the T10 segment. It is believed that although a person's brain can recognize that pain signals from the inflamed appendix are entering the spinal cord at the T10 segment, it interprets the pain signals to be emanating not from the visceral sensory nerve fibers that innervate the appendix but instead from the somatic sensory nerve fibers that innervate anterior abdominal wall tissues. Consequently, the patient experiences abdominal pain centered near the umbilicus, despite the fact that the pain signals are emanating from the appendix. Physicians label this altered perception of pain as referred pain, because the pain is referred to a site different from the site of origin of the pain signals.

In patients with acute appendicitis, the sign of RLQ quadrant tenderness upon deep palpation is present typically 12 to 24 hours after the onset of the diffuse periumbilical pain. By this time, the inflammatory process that has enveloped the appendix has extended to surrounding abdominal wall tissues, and it is these surrounding, inflamed abdominal wall tissues that emit somatic pain signals upon application of external pressure. "Whatever the constellation of signs and symptoms, the clinical diagnosis of acute appendicitis cannot be made unless tenderness (no matter how slight) can be demonstrated in some location."[3-4]

In patients with acute appendicitis, the symptom of a low-grade fever is also present typically 12 to 24 hours after the onset of the diffuse periumbilical pain. By this time, the patient's body is mounting a major inflammatory response to the inflamed appendix. Although nausea and anorexia are also common symptoms of acute appendicitis, each symptom is, in general and by itself, a non-specific symptom.

How then does a senior level medical student, upon consideration of the problem representation, conclude, rather quickly, that the most likely diagnosis is acute appendicitis? It is because in most medical schools today the curriculum addresses in some detail the most common diseases and injuries, and acute appendicitis is one of the most common diseases. In presenting the most common diseases and injuries, there is discussion of the most common signs and symptoms associated with each disease and injury. The set of the most common signs and symptoms that herald a disease or injury is referred to as the prototypical presentation of the disease or injury. The problem representation presented at the top of page 26 is a prototypical presentation of the signs and symptoms of acute appendicitis in a patient about 12 hours after the appearance of the periumbilical pain.

There are other important reasons why the prototypical presentation of acute appendicitis is almost universally discussed at some point in medical school. First and foremost, acute appendicitis is the most common pathophysiological cause of a syndrome known as the acute abdomen. The expression acute abdomen refers to any disease or injury that results in moderate to profound acute abdominal pain. The Research Committee of The World Organization of Gastroenterology conducted a study from 1978 to 1986 of over 10,000 cases of an acute abdomen in 30 hospitals, most of which were located in Europe and North America. Acute appendicitis was found to be the most common pathophysiological cause of an acute abdomen; it accounted for 28.1% of the cases.[3-5]

Second, the first principle of examining a person with an acute abdomen is "the necessity of making a serious and thorough attempt at diagnosis, usually predominantly by means of history and physical examination."[3-6] Diagnosis of an acute abdomen thus places a premium on the data acquired by the history and physical exam. Persons afflicted with an acute abdomen require prompt evaluation and frequently urgent treatment. There is always the risk that if the cause of an acute abdomen is not promptly and accurately diagnosed, the patient will suffer further complications or even succumb.

Third, even though there is general agreement on the prototypical presentations of an acute appendicitis at 12, 24, and 48 hours after the appearance of the periumbilical pain, it is also recognized that there is considerable variation in the actual presentations at each time interval. Much of this variability is due to the variable position of the appendix in the abdomen. Fig. 3-1 depicts the appendix hanging downward from the lower end of the right side of the large intestine; this is the position of the appendix that is commonly depicted in most anatomical atlases. However, in reality, the most common position of the appendix is the position in which the appendix lies posterior to, or behind, the lower end of the right side of the large intestine.[3-7] To further complicate matters, there is variation in the embryological development of the large intestine, which, in extreme cases, results in the appendix lying almost unbelievably in the left upper quadrant (LUQ) of the abdomen [the LUQ of the abdomen is the quarter of the abdomen above the umbilicus and to the left of the midline of the body].[3-8] "Many of the mistakes made in the diagnosis of appendicitis are due to a failure to realize the great difference in signs and symptoms that follow from the varying positions and relations of the appendix."[3-9]

A fourth and compelling reason why the prototypical presentation of acute appendicitis is almost universally discussed at some point in medical school is to demonstrate how difficult it is to accurately diagnose the acute abdomen syndrome in general. "Acute appendicitis can mimic virtually any intra-abdominal process; therefore, to know acute appendicitis is to know well the diagnosis of acute abdominal pain."[3-10] Diagnosis of the acute abdomen emphasizes an important feature of medical education today, namely, the significance of practicing evidence-based medicine (EBM) in the diagnosis and treatment of patients. With respect to diagnosis, EBM refers to the common practice today of physicians conducting control studies to assess the accuracy of a diagnostic test in detecting a target disorder. These control studies are important because when a diagnostic test is performed on a patient to detect a target disorder, it is necessary to understand that a positive test result does not necessarily imply that the patient has the disorder, and that, similarly, a negative test result does not necessarily imply that the patient does not have the disorder.

EBM studies of diagnostic tests are used to determine the sensitivity and specificity of the diagnostic tests. Whereas the sensitivity of a diagnostic test is the percentage of patients with the target disorder who test positive, the specificity of a diagnostic test is the percentage of patients without the target disorder who test negative. Physicians recognize that if a patient tests negative with a diagnostic test that has a high sensitivity, the negative result tends to rule out the diagnosis. This is because it is highly unlikely that a patient with the target disorder will test negative. Similarly, if a patient tests positive with a diagnostic test that has a high specificity, the positive result tends to rule in the diagnosis.

A critical feature of an EBM study of a diagnostic test is a procedure that establishes without any doubt that every patient enrolled in the study either had or did not have the target disorder. Such a procedure is called the "gold" standard; the "gold" standard is typically the findings of surgical exploration or a lab test result that does not require interpretation. The table below shows how the data acquired during an EBM study of a diagnostic test is used to calculate the sensitivity and specificity of the diagnostic test.

		TARGET DISORDER	
		PRESENT	ABSENT
DIAGNOSTIC TEST RESULT	POSITIVE	a	b
	NEGATIVE	c	d

a-NUMBER OF TRUE POSITIVE PATIENTS

b-NUMBER OF FALSE POSITIVE PATIENTS

c-NUMBER OF FALSE NEGATIVE PATIENTS

d-NUMBER OF TRUE NEGATIVE PATIENTS

$$\text{SENSITIVITY} = \frac{a}{a+c} = \text{PERCENTAGE OF PATIENTS WITH TARGET DISORDER WHO TEST POSITIVE}$$

$$\text{SPECIFICITY} = \frac{d}{b+d} = \text{PERCENTAGE OF PATIENTS WITHOUT TARGET DISORDER WHO TEST NEGATIVE}$$

There is no single diagnostic test that is commonly ordered for acute appendicitis. As has been noted, diagnosis is commonly made on the basis of the data acquired from the history, physical exam, and lab tests. The signs and symptoms almost always occur in the following order[3-11]:

1. Diffuse, dull pain around or near the umbilicus
2. Anorexia, nausea, or vomiting
3. Tenderness-somewhere in the abdomen or even the pelvis
4. Fever
5. Leukocytosis (increased white blood cell count)

If a patient presents with at least the first four findings in the order shown, physicians generally regard the aggregate of these four findings as the equivalent of a positive diagnostic test for acute appendicitis. Unless there is another possible diagnosis that merits examination, the patient undergoes immediate surgery. This is because an inflamed appendix is at very high risk of rupturing at some point 24 to 48 hours after the emergence of the dull, diffuse periumbilical pain. A ruptured, inflamed appendix releases bacteria throughout the peritoneal cavity of the abdomen and pelvis [the peritoneal cavity is a membrane-lined, fluid-filled cavity that extends throughout both the abdomen and pelvis and surrounds either partly or almost completely all the abdominal and pelvic organs]. Bacterial infection of the peritoneal cavity significantly complicates recovery of the patient and even places the patient's life at risk.

Of the patients who undergo appendectomy because of a common presentation for acute appendicitis, only about 80% are found to actually have acute appendicitis.[3-12] In other words, the sensitivity of regarding the aggregate of the above four or five findings as a diagnostic test for acute appendicitis is only about 80%.

Finally, it should be noted that in the study conducted by The Research Committee of The World Organization of Gastroenterology on over 10,000 cases of an acute abdomen, it was discovered that the most common 'cause' of an acute abdomen, and which accounted for 34% of the cases, was non-specific abdominal pain.[3-5] In other words, the abdominal pain in slightly more than one-third of the patients could not be attributed to any specific diagnosis. 34% of the patients had non-specific abdominal pain, 28.1% of the patients had acute appendicitis, and 9.7% of the patients had acute cholecystitis (acute inflammation of the gallbladder). Each of the remaining specific diagnoses accounted for 1.2 to 4.1% of the cases each.

It is very important now to mentally step back and reflect on what you have learned about the appendix and acute appendicitis in reading the preceding pages. It has been assumed that you, the reader, is a first-year medical student about to enter medical school or in the early part of your first semester in medical school. It has also been assumed that, unless you have suffered an acute appendicitis or known someone who had an acute appendicitis, you know little, if anything, about the appendix. Let's examine now what you have done or learned in reading the preceding pages:

1. You made your first attempt at constructing a problem representation, rich in semantic qualifiers, from a record of a patient's history and physical exam.

2. You learned the prototypical problem representation of a patient with an acute appendicitis when examined about 12 hours after the onset of periumbilical pain. Since the prototypical problem representation of a disease is the knowledge structure that mentally tags the illness script of the disease, you have completed the first cognitive step in creating your illness script for acute appendicitis.

3. You learned that the appendix is part of the large intestine, and you have a rough idea where it is generally found in the abdomen.

4. You learned that acute appendicitis is the condition in which the appendix becomes inflamed and swollen as a result of blockage of its lumen.

5. You learned the general definition of inflammation: it is the process by which the body recruits cells and factors from the blood to control and repair tissues damaged by disease or injury.

6. You learned that appendectomy is the only curative treatment of appendicitis.

7. You learned the definition of referred pain and the presumed rationale for its occurrence.

8. You learned that periumbilical pain is the first symptom to herald acute appendicitis and that it is an example of referred pain.

9. You learned that two semantic qualifiers of referred pain are that it is diffuse and dull.

10. You learned that nausea and anorexia are symptoms that individually are not specific for a particular diagnosis.

11. You learned that acute appendicitis is the most common pathophysiological cause of the acute abdomen syndrome.

12. You learned that diagnosis of an acute abdomen is derived mainly from the data acquired by the history and physical exam.

13. You learned that an acute abdomen must always be regarded initially as a life-threatening condition that requires prompt evaluation and possibly urgent treatment.

14. You learned that the clinical diagnosis of acute appendicitis cannot be made unless tenderness (no matter how slight) can be demonstrated in some location.

15. You learned that many of the mistakes made in the diagnosis of acute appendicitis are due to a failure to realize the great difference in signs and symptoms that follow from the varying positions and relations of the appendix.

16. You learned that EBM studies of a diagnostic test measure the sensitivity and specificity of the test and how the sensitivity and specificity are calculated from patient data.

17. You learned that if a patient tests negative with a diagnostic test that has a high sensitivity, the negative result tends to rule out the diagnosis. Similarly, if a patient tests positive with a diagnostic test that has a high specificity, the positive result tends to rule in the diagnosis.

18.   You learned that the generally accepted positive diagnostic test for acute appendicitis is the appearance of four findings in a specific order, and that this test has a sensitivity of about 80%.

19.   Finally, you learned that it is not be possible to designate a specific diagnosis for about one-third of all the patients examined for an acute abdomen.

Observe that all of everything you either did or learned as you read the preceding pages was done or learned in relation to the clinical findings of patients who present with signs and symptoms suggestive of acute appendicitis. There was no detailed discussion of the embryological development, microscopic anatomy, gross anatomy, physiology, or immunological characterization of the appendix. In other words, even though you now know as much if not more about the clinical presentation of acute appendicitis than any graduating fourth-year medical student, you were able to learn all this material in the absence of any of the basic medical science knowledge about the appendix that you will be exposed to during your first 18 to 24 months in medical school.

The implication of having learned about acute appendicitis before you learn basic medical science knowledge about the appendix is profound. This is because as you learn basic medical science knowledge about the appendix, you will be embedding that knowledge in your illness script for acute appendicitis. This is exactly how Flexner argued that basic medical science knowledge should be learned in medical school. It is also exactly how Knowles' theory of adult learning and contemporary theories of cognitive psychology suggest is the most practical way of learning basic medical science knowledge in medical school. Consequently, starting 18 to 24 months from now, the first time you encounter a patient with a problem representation that activates your recall of the illness script for acute appendicitis, that cue will also activate in your memory what you learned about the embryological development, microscopic anatomy, gross anatomy, physiology, and immunological characterization of the appendix.

We can now discuss the first three measures you can take during your first 18 to 24 months in medical school to learn the basic medical sciences in relation to the clinical findings of patients. First, whenever you are presented with any opportunity either to study a record of a patient's history and physical exam or to watch the history and physical exam of a real or standardized patient, attempt to identify as many of the semantic qualifiers of the patient's signs and symptoms as you can [a standardized patient is an otherwise healthy person who has been trained to assume the role of a person afflicted with a specific disease or injury]. Second, if given the opportunity, attempt to construct a problem representation of the patient's condition that includes as many as possible of the semantic qualifiers. You should now appreciate that, in attempting to conduct these two cognitive steps, you are progressively perfecting the first two cognitive steps you will always take as you attempt to diagnose a patient's condition.

Third, maintain a record of prototypical problem representations of common diseases and injuries that are presented to you in the course of your basic medical science studies. You now know that these prototypical problem representations serve as the diagnostic tags of the illness scripts of these diseases and injuries. Attempt to populate each illness script with data regarding factors that predispose a person to the disease or injury and the pathophysiological mechanism that accounts for the signs and symptoms of the disease or injury. This is important because, as will be discussed in the following chapter, illness scripts are not merely cognitive structures that facilitate diagnosis, but, more importantly, serve as story lines that help physicians understand why a person may be more prone to a disease or injury and the mechanism by which a disease or an injury occurs.

REFERENCES

3-1. Bordage G. Prototypes and Semantic Qualifiers: from Past to Present. Medical Education (2007) 41:1171-1121.

3-2. Fleming A, Cutrer W, Reimschisel T, and J Gigante. You Too Can Teach Clinical Reasoning! Pediatrics (2012) 130:795-797.

3-3. Bowen, JL. Educational Strategies to Promote Clinical Diagnostic Reasoning. New England Journal of Medicine (2006) 355:2217-2225 p. 2218.

3-4. Silen, W. Cope's Early Diagnosis of the Acute Abdomen. 22nd edition. (2010) Oxford University Press. p. 73.

3-5. de Dombal, FT. Diagnosis of Acute Abdominal Pain (1991) Churchill Livingstone. p. 20.

3-6. Silen, W. Cope's Early Diagnosis of the Acute Abdomen. 22nd edition. (2010) Oxford University Press. p. 3.

3-7. Slaby, FJ. The Clinically Oriented Gross Anatomy Lab Workbook. (2010) On-Demand Publishing. p. 190.

3-8. Silen, W. Cope's Early Diagnosis of the Acute Abdomen. 22nd edition. (2010) Oxford University Press. p. 69.

3-9. Silen, W. Cope's Early Diagnosis of the Acute Abdomen. 22nd edition. (2010) Oxford University Press. p. 70.

3-10. Silen, W. Cope's Early Diagnosis of the Acute Abdomen. 22nd edition. (2010) Oxford University Press. p. 84.

3-11. Silen, W. Cope's Early Diagnosis of the Acute Abdomen. 22nd edition. (2010) Oxford University Press. p. 76.

3-12. http://radiology.rsna.org/content/215/2/337.full

Chapter 4

ILLNESS SCRIPTS AND INSTANCE SCRIPTS

You learned in the previous chapter that experienced physicians develop cognitive structures called illness scripts in which are embedded not only the pathophysiology of diseases and injuries but also the conditions that predispose a person to the diseases and injuries. You also learned that problem representations serve as the diagnostic tags of illness scripts. In this chapter we will examine more thoroughly the structure of illness scripts and how experienced physicians develop and use them and further differentiate them into instance scripts.

Feltovich and Barrows were the first investigators of medical problem solving to propose that physicians structure their medical knowledge in scripts.[4-1] Charlin et al. have described the script concept as follows:

"The basic principle underpinning the script concept asserts that, to give meaning to a new situation in our environment, we use prior knowledge that contains information about the characteristics and features of the situation and information about the relationships that link those characteristics and features. In other words, incoming information activates a previously acquired network of relevant knowledge and experience-a *script*-that directs the selection, interpretation, and memorization of that new information. In medicine, when a physician sees a patient, he or she perceives features-symptoms, signs, and details from the patient's environment-that activate networks of knowledge that contain those features and their relationships to illnesses. These networks of knowledge then provide context, and thus meaning, to the new situation."[4-2]

Illness scripts are scripts of medical knowledge designed to provide efficient and accurate diagnosis. The illness scripts of an experienced physician are highly personalized cognitive structures that are developed and reiteratively refined during several years of examining patients.[4-3] Consequently, if, for example, a group of experienced primary care physicians were asked to describe their illness script for asthma, one would find a broad consensus on certain features and yet variable differences on other features. Illness scripts thus exhibit an idiosyncratic nature that is always subject to further differentiation upon examination of future patients.

The illness scripts of experienced physicians have a generic, tripartite structure (Fig. 4-1).[4-4] In the mind of an experienced physician, every illness script tells a story. The story begins with the sex and other genetic factors with which a patient was born and continues with the lifestyle habits that the patient adopts. These are the enabling conditions. The critical event in the story is the fault, that is, the occurrence of a disease or an injury. Experienced physicians regard the enabling conditions as factors that increased the likelihood of the occurrence of the fault. For example, cigarette smoking is regarded as a factor that predisposes a person to chronic obstructive pulmonary disease (COPD), a disease that affects the airways of the lungs. Similarly, lifelong tennis players are prone to injury of the rotator cuff muscles of the shoulder, as these muscles are subject to considerable stress when a player serves the ball. Finally, the fault produces the complaints, symptoms, and signs of the patient.

Observe in the figure of the generic illness script that the information in each of the three main parts of the script appears to be compartmentalized in slots. The information contained in each of these slots is called an attribute of the illness script.

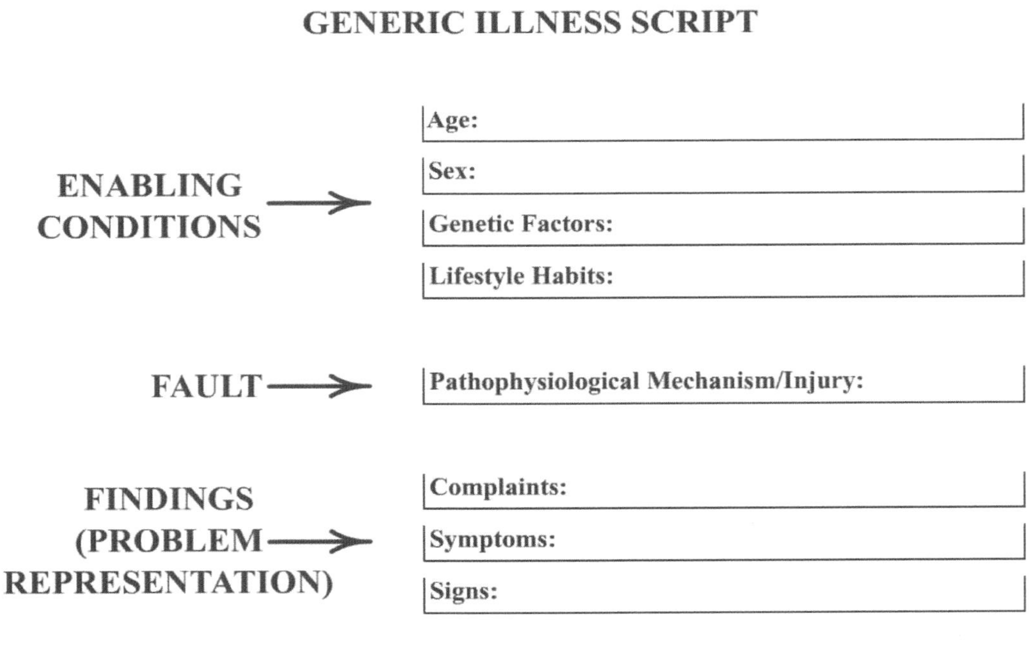

GENERIC ILLNESS SCRIPT

ENABLING CONDITIONS ⟶
- Age:
- Sex:
- Genetic Factors:
- Lifestyle Habits:

FAULT ⟶
- Pathophysiological Mechanism/Injury:

FINDINGS (PROBLEM ⟶ REPRESENTATION)
- Complaints:
- Symptoms:
- Signs:

Fig. 4-1: The tripartite structure of a generic illness script.

Observe that an experienced physician's illness scripts each provide two contrasting views of the fault: (1) the conditions and factors that increase the likelihood of the fault occurring and (2) the consequences of the fault. This dual perspective benefits the diagnostic skills of an experienced physician in three ways. First, it gives the experienced physician a more realistic understanding of the nature of diseases and injuries. Diseases and injuries are not random events that may occur with equal likelihood in any person. There are conditions and factors, some of which a person can control and others which a person cannot control, that either contribute to or protect against the occurrence of a disease or injury.[4-5]

Second, the dual perspective provides a more comprehensive view of the pathophysiological mechanism of a disease or the mechanical nature of an injury. An experienced physician can explain not only how the pathophysiological mechanism of a disease results in a patient's symptoms and signs, but also how the enabling conditions lead to the initiation of the pathophysiological mechanism.

Third, the dual perspective offers the experienced physician two diagnostic pathways. In the early years of an experienced physician's training (that is, the medical school, residency, and early clinical practice years), a physician diagnoses almost exclusively via his/her analysis of the problem representation of a patient, which highlights the patient's complaints, symptoms, and signs. There is evidence that as a physician in clinical practice increasingly acquires diagnostic experience, he/she increasingly relies on a patient's enabling conditions and factors to identify efficiently and effectively the illness script which most closely describes the patient's condition.[4-6, 4-7, 4-8] In other words, as physicians increasingly acquire diagnostic experience, they ascribe two diagnostic tags to a patient's illness script: the problem representation of the patient's condition and, what could be termed, the predisposed representation of the patient's condition.

In order to clarify how a physician develops an illness script for one of the diseases and/or injuries in his/her field of specialty, let's consider how an emergency medicine physician develops an illness script for acute cholecystitis. You will recall from the previous chapter that acute cholecystitis is inflammation of the gallbladder, and that acute cholecystitis is the second most common cause of an acute abdomen. In order to understand the common etiology of acute cholecystitis, we need first to discuss the gross anatomy of the gallbladder, its role in the digestive system, and the most common cause of acute cholecystitis.

The gallbladder is a pear-shaped sac that lies suspended from the lower part of the posterior surface of the liver. The lower end of the gallbladder is called its fundus; the fundus is the expanded, blind end of the gallbladder (Fig. 4-2). The upper end of the gallbladder is called its neck; the neck is the narrowed, open end of the gallbladder. The region of the gallbladder between its fundus and neck is called the body of the gallbladder. The duct that extends from the neck of the gallbladder is called the cystic duct.

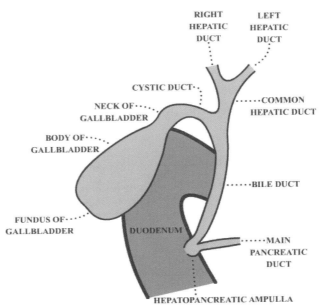

Fig. 4-2: The gallbladder and its relationships with the ducts that conduct bile from the liver to the duodenum.

The cystic duct communicates with the biliary ducts that conduct bile from the liver and gallbladder to the duodenum. The duodenum is the first segment of the small intestine; it receives foodstuffs that have been partially digested in the stomach. The liver continuously produces bile that exits the liver via two ducts called the left and right hepatic ducts. The left and right hepatic ducts unite to form the common hepatic duct, which in turn unites with the cystic duct to form the bile duct. In the wall of the duodenum, the bile duct unites with the main pancreatic duct to form a short but bulbous duct called the hepatopancreatic ampulla. A sphincter called the hepatopancreatic sphincter surrounds the opening of the hepatopancreatic ampulla into the lumen (that is, the interior) of the duodenum.

Sphincter of Oddi

40

During fasting periods, the hepatopancreatic sphincter is closed shut. Fasting periods are the periods between meals when nutrients are no longer being absorbed by the small intestine. Consequently, during fasting periods, bile newly produced by the liver drains via the hepatic ducts into first the bile duct, and after the bile duct is completely filled with bile, the bile next drains into the cystic duct and gallbladder. During fasting periods, the gallbladder serves to store and concentrate bile.

After a meal, the passage of partially digested food from the stomach into the duodenum stimulates certain endocrine cells within the wall of the duodenum to secrete a polypeptide hormone called cholecystokinin (CCK) into the blood circulation. The blood circulation carries the CCK to the duodenum, the gallbladder, and the pancreas. In the duodenum, CCK relaxes the smooth muscle cells of the hepatopancreatic sphincter, and thus the sphincter opens. In the gallbladder, CCK stimulates rhythmic contractions of the smooth muscle cells in the wall of the gallbladder. These contractions expel concentrated bile into the lumen of the duodenum. In the pancreas, CCK stimulates the secretion of digestive enzymes into pancreatic juice. The pancreatic juice enters the lumen of the duodenum mixed with bile. Pancreatic juice is rich in a wide variety of enzymes that digest complex carbohydrates into simpler sugars, proteins into small polypeptides and amino acids, and fats into fatty acids. The bile acids in bile greatly aid first in the emulsification, or physical break-up, of fats in foodstuffs and later the enzymatic digestion of fats into fatty acids.

The event that evokes acute cholecystitis in 90% of all cases is the entrapment of a gallstone in the cystic duct. If the cystic duct obstruction persists for more than a few hours, acute inflammation of the wall of the gallbladder begins. The medical term for gallstone formation is cholelithiasis. Gallstones develop insidiously and may be asymptomatic throughout most of adulthood. Gallstones develop as a result of precipitation and progressive crystallization of either cholesterol or calcium bilirubinate in the bile. Bilirubin is a product of the breakdown of the heme groups in hemoglobin molecules.

Now that you know the role of the gallbladder in the digestive system and the most common cause of acute cholecystitis, let's examine the illness script that an intern (that is, a first-year resident) in an emergency medicine residency constructs upon her first examination in her medical career of a patient, a 40 year-old male, with acute cholecystitis. Upon examining the patient, the intern constructs the following problem representation: The patient is a 40 year-old febrile, anorexic, nauseated male with diffuse, dull, unrelenting RUQ pain of 4 hours duration. Physical examination elicits a positive Murphy's sign. The patient undergoes a cholecystectomy (surgical removal of the gallbladder) following ultrasonographic evidence for the presence of gallstones and indication of an enlarged, inflamed gallbladder.

The physical exam maneuver for detecting Murphy's sign begins with the patient lying supine upon an examination table. The examiner curls his/her fingertips under the midregion of the right costal margin of the patient's rib cage and then asks the patient to take a deep breath (Fig. 4-3). As the patient's takes a deep breath, the descent of the diaphragm pushes the liver and the gallbladder downward together within the abdomen. If the gallbladder is inflamed, the pressing of the fundus of the swollen gallbladder against the examiner's fingertips suddenly elicits increased pain and abrupt cessation of breathing by the patient. Abrupt cessation of breathing in is called inspiratory arrest. Inspiratory arrest and/or complaint by the patient of enhanced pain represents a positive Murphy's sign.

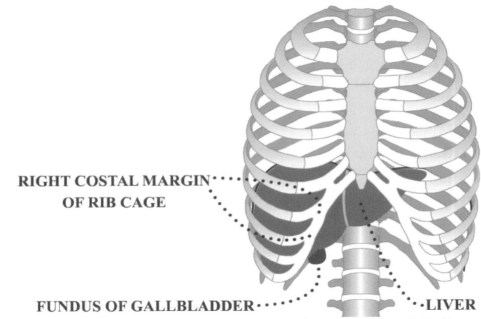

RIGHT COSTAL MARGIN
OF RIB CAGE

FUNDUS OF GALLBLADDER · · · · · · · · · · · · · · LIVER

Fig. 4-3: The relationships of the anterior-inferior margin of the liver and the fundus of the gallbladder relative to the right costal margin of the rib cage.

Upon confirming from the surgeon that the 40 year-old male was indeed suffering from acute cholecystitis, the emergency medicine intern mentally constructs an illness script for the disease specific to that patient (the top script in Fig. 4-4). An illness script specific to a patient is called an instance script. During the next 5 years the physician encounters in her residency and early medical practice 39 more patients with surgically-confirmed acute cholecystitis. At each encounter, the physician subconsciously incorporates the specifics of each instance script into a progressively changing general illness script for the disease, whose attributes after 40 patients are as shown in the bottom script in Fig. 4-4. The attributes of the problem representation have changed substantially. The physician has learned that the acute, unrelenting pain can occasionally be better described as being in the epigastric region of the abdomen as opposed to the RUQ. Physicians sometimes divide the abdomen into 9 regions instead of 4 quadrants (Fig. 4-5). In dividing the abdomen into 9 equal regions, two vertical planes passing through the midpoints of the patient's clavicles intersect two horizontal planes. The darkened, uppermost central region depicted in Fig. 4-5 is called the epigastric region because it lies immediately superior to the pyloric region of the stomach.

The physician has also learned that although the acute, unrelenting RUQ/epigastric pain of acute cholecystitis is commonly accompanied by fever and leukocytosis, either or both of these two latter signs may be absent.[4-9] She recognizes that the extremely high sensitivity (97%) of Murphy's sign implies that if a patient with suspected acute cholecystitis tests negative for Murphy's sign, it is likely that the patient is not suffering from acute cholecystitis.[4-10] She has also encountered patients in which the pain of acute cholecystitis radiated to the interscapular area of the back (the area between the scapulae), the right scapula, or the right shoulder.

The attributes of the enabling conditions and factors have also changed. The physician has found, as would be predicted on statistical grounds, that most patients are women.[4-11] The physician has also found that, in contrast to her first patient, most patients present with a history of biliary colic.[4-10] Biliary colic is the pain that is produced when a gallstone enters or passes through the cystic duct or common bile duct. "The term biliary colic is essentially a misnomer, since the pain arising from the passage of a biliary stone is steady and not paroxysmal."[4-12] The pain of biliary colic "varies considerably in intensity, depending on how hard it is for the stone to traverse the ducts, and is usually sudden in onset and severe in intensity."[4-12] The pain of biliary colic is very similar in its nature and location to the pain heralding acute cholecystitis. The physician thus recognizes that "the usual attack of acute cholecystitis begins with an episode of biliary colic."[4-13] In a patient suffering from biliary colic, acute cholecystitis becomes suspect when the biliary colic-type pain lasts for more than 4 to 6 hours and a positive Murphy's sign or RUQ tenderness to deep palpation is encountered.

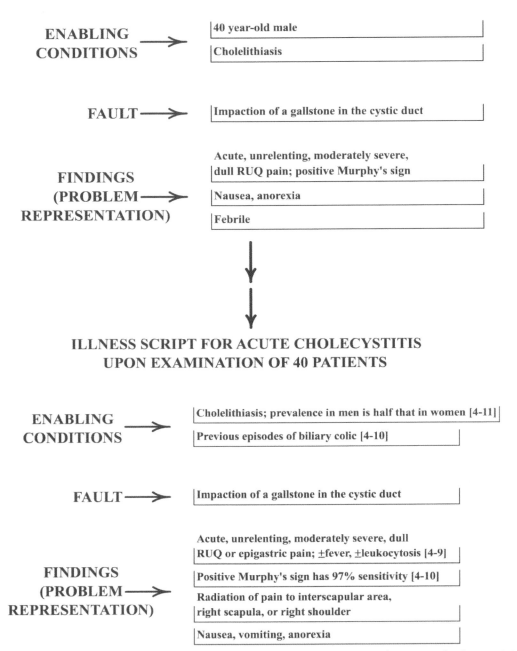

INSTANCE ILLNESS SCRIPT
FOR THE FIRST PATIENT
WITH ACUTE CHOLECYSTITIS

ENABLING CONDITIONS →

40 year-old male

Cholelithiasis

FAULT →

Impaction of a gallstone in the cystic duct

FINDINGS (PROBLEM REPRESENTATION) →

Acute, unrelenting, moderately severe, dull RUQ pain; positive Murphy's sign

Nausea, anorexia

Febrile

ILLNESS SCRIPT FOR ACUTE CHOLECYSTITIS
UPON EXAMINATION OF 40 PATIENTS

ENABLING CONDITIONS →

Cholelithiasis; prevalence in men is half that in women [4-11]

Previous episodes of biliary colic [4-10]

FAULT →

Impaction of a gallstone in the cystic duct

FINDINGS (PROBLEM REPRESENTATION) →

Acute, unrelenting, moderately severe, dull RUQ or epigastric pain; ±fever, ±leukocytosis [4-9]

Positive Murphy's sign has 97% sensitivity [4-10]

Radiation of pain to interscapular area, right scapula, or right shoulder

Nausea, vomiting, anorexia

Fig 4-4: The elaboration of a physician's first instance script of acute cholecystitis into a general illness script following the examination of 40 patients with the disease.

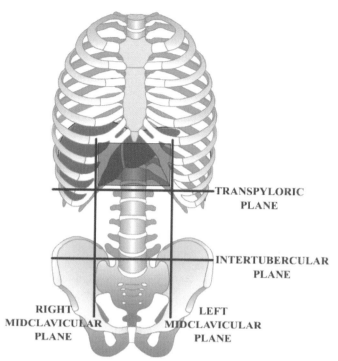

Fig. 4-5: The division of the abdomen into 9 equivalent regions. The transpyloric plane lies at the level of the pyloric region of the stomach; the pyloric region is the end region of the stomach. The intertubercular plane lies at the level of the prominent enlargements along the upper margins of the hip bones; the enlargements are called the tubercles. The darkened region is the epigastric region.

Recognition that highly experienced physicians can employ both a problem representation and a predisposed representation of a patient's condition to diagnose a patient's condition brings us to the point at which we can now discuss what is known about how highly experienced physicians conduct diagnosis. By definition, a highly experienced physician is a physician who, in his/her field of medical expertise, can efficiently identify an accurate or most likely diagnosis of a patient's condition.

In their field of expertise, highly experienced physicians typically begin identifying possible illness scripts relatively early in the taking of the patient's history (Fig. 4-6). Acquiring information about a few of the patient's findings is frequently sufficient to activate in the physician's mind selection of at least one illness script. At this moment, the physician typically redirects his/her questions to topics whose answers will provide further information on certain enabling conditions or patient findings in the selected illness script. The physician is thus applying at this juncture hypothetical-deductive reasoning. In selecting a specific illness script, the physician has, in effect, hypothesized that this is the illness script that identifies the patient's condition. The physician then deduces that, if this hypothesis is correct, the patient's answers to my next questions should match certain enabling conditions or findings of the selected illness script. If the patient's answers match or are compatible with the information in the selected illness script, the physician may ask 1 or 2 more questions. If once again, the patient's answers again match or are compatible with the information in the selected illness script, the physician arrives at a "saturation point" and concludes that the most likely diagnosis has been identified.[4-14]

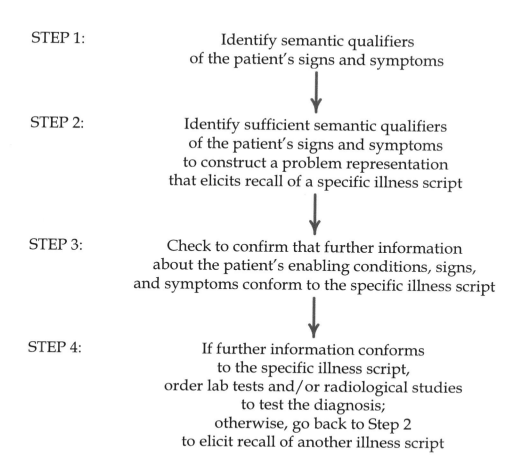

STEP 1:   Identify semantic qualifiers
of the patient's signs and symptoms

STEP 2:   Identify sufficient semantic qualifiers
of the patient's signs and symptoms
to construct a problem representation
that elicits recall of a specific illness script

STEP 3:   Check to confirm that further information
about the patient's enabling conditions, signs,
and symptoms conform to the specific illness script

STEP 4:   If further information conforms
to the specific illness script,
order lab tests and/or radiological studies
to test the diagnosis;
otherwise, go back to Step 2
to elicit recall of another illness script

Fig. 4-6: Common cognitive diagnostic steps by which an experienced physician conducts diagnosis in his/her field of expertise.

In a nutshell, this then is one of the essential differences in diagnostic skills between medical students and experienced physicians: Experienced physicians have a multitude of highly-detailed illness scripts in their field of expertise, and each of these illness scripts has two diagnostic tags: its problem representation and its predisposed representation. Medical students have a sparse number of partly-defined illness scripts representative of all the fields of medicine, and each of these illness scripts has only one diagnostic tag: its problem representation.

The essential difference in the utility of illness scripts between medical students and experienced physicians thus boils down to just one thing: experience. This is why it is important here to repeat the advice offered at the end of the previous chapter: During your first 18 to 24 months in medical school, take full advantage of every opportunity to:

(1) view or read about a patient's history and physical exam,

(2) identify the semantic qualifiers of the patient's signs and symptoms,

(3) construct a problem representation, heavily populated with semantic qualifiers, of the patient's condition, and

(4) construct a tripartite-structured illness script that identifies any enabling conditions and factors, the mechanism of the patient's disease or injury, and the complaints, symptoms, and signs of the patient at the time of his/her examination.

This habit of constructing illness scripts of real and fictional patients is not just a prudent study habit. This is because every time you construct an illness script of a real or fictional patient, you are constructing an instance script. It should be evident at this juncture of your reading of this book that any time an experienced physician examines a patient, the physician, in effect, also constructs an instance script.[4-15] An experienced physician diagnoses a patient's condition by basically comparing and contrasting the patient's instance script with the physician's catalogue of illness scripts. Numerous studies have demonstrated that physicians can recall the instance scripts of certain patients many years after the patients were examined.

Consequently, by adopting the habit of constructing illness scripts of real and fictional patients during your first 18 to 24 months in medical school, you are, in effect, assembling a catalogue of instance scripts. Even if all the instance scripts pertain to fictional patients, they are still highly relevant. This is because when your instructors present a fictional patient, they commonly imbue the patient with prototypical enabling conditions, complaints, signs, and symptoms of a specific disease or injury. The instructors also tend to highlight in these fictional patients the most common or most significant diseases and injuries that afflict the American population, such as coronary artery disease, hypertension, asthma, COPD, insulin-dependent or non-insulin-dependent diabetes, thyroid disease, various types of cancer, AIDS, various types of arthritis, depression, and dementia. The instance script that you develop for any of these conditions is simply the first rendition of the illness script for that condition that you will continue to refine as you proceed through medical school, residency, and clinical practice.

The two most important benefits of adopting the habit of constructing illness scripts of real and fictional patients during your first 18 to 24 months in medical school are that you are (1) practicing and refining from your first days in medical school one of the cognitive diagnostic skill sets of experienced physicians and (2) imposing a complaint-based scheme (as opposed to a discipline-based scheme) on the organization of your basic medical science knowledge. By knowing, from your first days in medical school, the roles that data acquisition, hypothetical-deductive reasoning, semantic qualifiers, problems representations, illness scripts, and instance scripts play in the diagnostic practices of experienced physicians, you can begin medical school by emulating these practices and taking the initiative in not only developing your diagnostic reasoning skills but also organizing your basic medical science knowledge in relation to the clinical findings of patients.

REFERENCES

4-1. Feltovich PJ and HS Barrows. Issues of Generality in Medical Problem Solving. In: Schmidt HG and ML DeVolder eds. Tutorials in Problem-Based Learning. Assen / Maastricht: Van Gorcum (1984) pp. 128–142.

4-2. Charlin B, Tardif J, and H Boshuizen. Scripts and Medical Knowledge: Theory and Applications for Clinical Reasoning Instruction and Research. Academic Medicine (2000) 75:182-190. p. 183.

4-3. Schmidt HG, Norman GR, and HPA Boshuizen. A Cognitive Perspective on Medical Expertise: Theory and Implications. Academic Medicine (1990) 65:611-621 p. 617.

4-4. Schmidt HG, Norman GR, and HPA Boshuizen. A Cognitive Perspective on Medical Expertise: Theory and Implications. Academic Medicine (1990) 65:611-621 p. 615.

4-5. Charlin B, Boshuizen HPA, Custers, EJ, and PJ Feltovich, Illness Scripts and Clinical Reasoning. Medical Education (2007) 41:1178-1184. p. 1181.

4-6. Schmidt HG, Norman GR, and HPA Boshuizen. A Cognitive Perspective on Medical Expertise: Theory and Implications. Academic Medicine (1990) 65:611-621 p. 616.

4-7. Hobus PPM, Hofstra ML, Boshuizen HPA, and HG Schmidt. The Context of A Complaint As A Diagnostic Tool. Huisarts en Wetenschap (1988) 31:261-267.

4-8. Schmidt HG and RMJP Rikers. How Expertise Develops in Medicine: Knowledge Encapsulation and Illness Script Formation. Medical Education (2007) 41:1133-1139 p. 1137.

4-9.   Strasberg SM.   Acute Calculous Cholecystitis.   New England Journal of Medicine (2008) 358:2804-2811 p. 2805.

4-10. Yusoff IF, Barkun JS, and AN Barkun.   Diagnosis and Management of Cholecystitis and Cholangitis.   Gastroenterology Clinics of North America (2003) 32:1145-1168 p. 1146.

4-11. Strasberg SM. Acute Calculous Cholecystitis. New England Journal of Medicine (2008) 358:2804-2811 p. 2804.

4-12. Silen, W. Cope's Early Diagnosis of the Acute Abdomen. 22nd edition. (2010) Oxford University Press. p. 149.

4-13. Silen, W. Cope's Early Diagnosis of the Acute Abdomen. 22nd edition. (2010) Oxford University Press. p. 132.

4-14. Bonilauri Ferreira APR, Ferreira RF, Rajgor D, Shah J, Menezes A, et al. Clinical Reasoning in the Real World Is Mediated by Bounded Rationality: Implications for Diagnostic Clinical Practice Guidelines. (2010) PLoS ONE 5(4): e10265. doi:10.1371/journal.pone.0010265. pp. 4 and 5.

4-15. Schmidt HG, Norman GR, and HPA Boshuizen. A Cognitive Perspective on Medical Expertise: Theory and Implications. Academic Medicine (1990) 65:611-621 p. 617.

Chapter 5

SCHEME-INDUCTIVE REASONING

At this point in our discussion of the cognitive basis of diagnostic reasoning, you should now appreciate that when you are challenged to consider a patient's history and physical exam findings in one of your clinical clerkships, you begin your analysis by first identifying the semantic qualifiers of the patient's complaints, signs and symptoms and next incorporating them into a succinct problem representation of the patient's condition. You should also now appreciate that if you were an experienced physician, you would compare and contrast the patient's problem representation with those of similar illness scripts or instance scripts in an attempt to identify the most likely diagnosis. However, as a third-year or fourth-year medical student, you will most likely have only a limited register of illness scripts and instance scripts. What, then, is an effective approach in the clinical clerkships for developing clinical reasoning skills beyond the cognitive steps of semantic qualifiers and problem representations?

There is evidence from medical education research that scheme-inductive reasoning is an effective approach. The first medical school to organize its curriculum around scheme-inductive reasoning was the University of Calgary Faculty of Medicine in Calgary, Alberta, Canada, in the early 1990's. Their innovation was based on the following assumption: "The manner or mode in which the human body reacts to an infinite number of insults is finite and stable over time. The modes in which patients present to physicians [is to be] termed *clinical presentations*, defined as the common and important ways in which a person, group of people, community, or population present to a physician. These modes represent problems that a graduating physician is expected to manage."[5-1] The Calgary faculty identified over 120 clinical presentations. The following list illustrates the comprehensive nature of the clinical presentations they identified:

Amenorrhea (abnormal absence of menstruation)

Anemia

Chest Discomfort

Chronic Abdominal Pain (Adult)

Diffuse Lymphadenopathy (dispersed, enlarged lymph nodes)

Dysphagia (difficulty swallowing)

Fatigue

Fever and Chills

Hypertension

Primary Skin Lesions
Psychotic Disorders
Sore Throat
Splenomegaly (enlarged spleen)
Suspected DVT (suspicion of Deep Venous Thrombi [blood clots] in the legs)
Syncope (temporary loss of consciousness)

In order to assist their students in organizing their thoughts about the pathophysiological mechanisms or injuries that could be responsible for each of the clinical presentations, the faculty developed schemes to aid diagnostic reasoning. A complete list of the clinical presentations and the scheme or schemes that assist diagnosis of each clinical presentation can be accessed at the following website: http://www.scribd.com/doc/53149012/Calgary-Black-Book. The guidelines that the faculty followed in developing the schemes are described at the website and presented as follows:

"There is no single right way to approach any given clinical presentation. Each of the schemes provided represents one approach that proved useful and meaningful to one experienced, expert author. A modified, personalized scheme may be better than someone else's scheme, and certainly better than having no scheme at all. It is important to keep in mind, before creating a scheme, the five fundamentals of scheme creation that were used in the development of this book. If a scheme is to be useful the answers to the next five questions should be positive:

1. Is it simple and easy to remember? (does is reduce memory load by 'chunking' information into categories and subcategories)

2. Does it provide an organizational structure that is easy to alter?

3. Does the organizing principle of the scheme enhance the meaning of the information?

4. Does the organizing principle of the scheme mirror encoding specificity? (both context and process specificity)

5. Does the scheme aid in problem solving? (e.g. does it differentiate between large categories initially, and subsequently progressively smaller ones until a single diagnosis is reached)"

The decision by the Calgary faculty to develop a curriculum based on clinical presentations and diagnostic schemes is in accordance with the tenets of Knowles' theory of adult learning and Flexner's admonition that the basic medical sciences should be learned in relation to the clinical findings of patients. Another Canadian medical school, McMaster's School of Medicine in Hamilton, Ontario, undertook a similar initiative when the school developed a problem-based learning (PBL) curriculum at its founding in 1966. PBL promotes self-directed learning by medical students as they attempt to learn basic medical science content in the context of individual cases.

In Calgary's curriculum, each clinical presentation is named for a symptom, a sign, or a lab test result that characterizes a patient's condition. The clinical presentation is thus a specific, abnormal finding of the patient's health. In order to demonstrate how a diagnostic scheme facilitates analysis of a clinical presentation, let us consider a specific clinical presentation: dyspnea. Dyspnea is difficulty in breathing. The diagnostic scheme for dyspnea presented here (Fig. 5-1) has been adapted and simplified from the scheme for dyspnea at Calgary's website. The dyspnea scheme in Fig. 5-1 focuses on dyspnea that is only either of cardiac origin or pulmonary origin. If the dyspnea is of cardiac origin, the scheme identifies three major categories of cardiac dysfunction that can lead to dyspnea. If the dyspnea is of pulmonary origin, the scheme identifies three major categories of pulmonary structure and function whose dysfunction can lead to dyspnea.

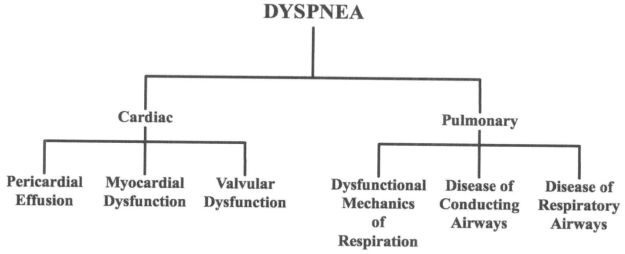

Fig. 5-1: Diagnostic scheme for dyspnea.

In order to appreciate how a third-year or fourth-year medical student would use this diagnostic scheme for dyspnea in the analysis of a patient's condition, we need first to clarify why cardiac dysfunction, in general, can lead to dyspnea.

The heart is a hollowed-out organ with a left side and a right side (Fig. 5-2). Each side has two chambers, a smaller one called an atrium and a larger one called a ventricle. The two chambers on the right side are called the right atrium and right ventricle, and two chambers on the left side are called the left atrium and left ventricle. Whereas the atria are the chambers that receive blood on each side of the heart, the ventricles are the chambers that eject blood from each side of the heart.

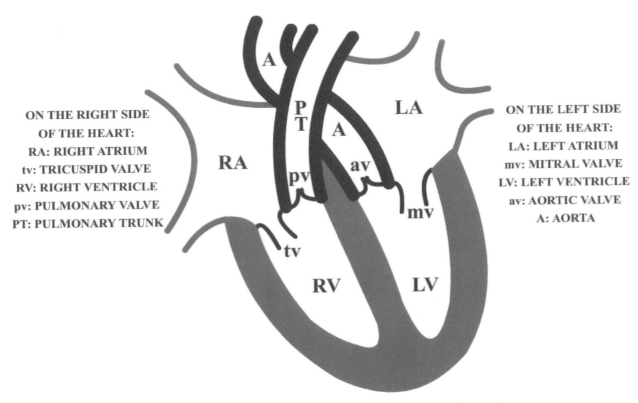

ON THE RIGHT SIDE
OF THE HEART:
RA: RIGHT ATRIUM
tv: TRICUSPID VALVE
RV: RIGHT VENTRICLE
pv: PULMONARY VALVE
PT: PULMONARY TRUNK

ON THE LEFT SIDE
OF THE HEART:
LA: LEFT ATRIUM
mv: MITRAL VALVE
LV: LEFT VENTRICLE
av: AORTIC VALVE
A: AORTA

Fig. 5-2: Coronal section of the heart during diastole:
whereas the tricuspid and mitral valves are open;
the pulmonary and aortic valves are closed.

The right atrium receives oxygen-poor blood from the body's tissues, and the right ventricle ejects the oxygen-poor blood toward the lungs via a large artery called the pulmonary trunk; a valve called the pulmonary valve guards the opening of the right ventricle into the pulmonary trunk (Fig. 5-2). The left atrium receives oxygen-rich blood from the lungs, and the left ventricle ejects the oxygen-rich blood throughout the body via a large artery called the aorta; a valve called the aortic valve guards the opening of the left ventricle into the aorta.

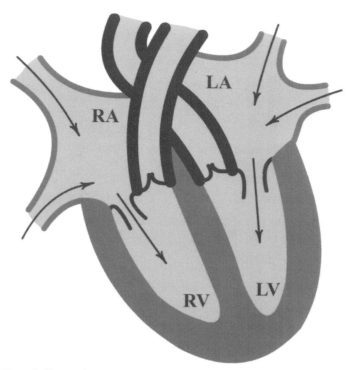

Fig. 5-3: Blood flow through the heart's chambers during diastole.

Each heartbeat can be described by a single cycle of events called the cardiac cycle. The cardiac cycle begins with a period called diastole, during which all the heart muscle tissue in the walls of the left and right ventricles is relaxed (Fig. 5-3). On the right side of the heart throughout diastole, the right atrium receives oxygen-poor blood that has been drained from the body's tissues and conducts the blood into the right ventricle. A valve called the tricuspid valve guards the opening of the right atrium into the right ventricle; the tricuspid valve is open throughout diastole. On the left side of the heart throughout diastole, the left atrium receives oxygen-rich blood from the lungs and conducts the blood into the left ventricle. A valve called the mitral valve guards the opening of the left atrium into the left ventricle. Like the tricuspid valve, the mitral valve is open throughout diastole. The pulmonary and aortic valves are closed throughout diastole.

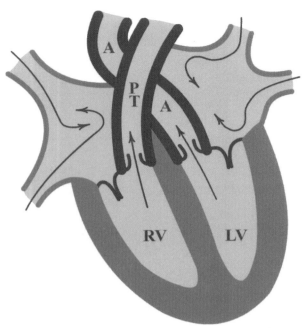

Fig. 5-4: Blood is ejected from the right ventricle into the pulmonary trunk and from the left ventricle into the aorta during systole. Blood continues to flow into the atria during systole.

The cardiac cycle ends with a period called systole, during which all the heart muscle tissue in the ventricles contracts. On the right side of the heart during systole, the rapid increase in blood pressure in the right ventricle quickly closes the tricuspid valve and then forces open the pulmonary valve to eject oxygen-poor blood toward the lungs (Fig. 5-4). On the left side of the heart during systole, the rapid increase in blood pressure in the left ventricle quickly closes the mitral valve and then forces open the aortic valve to eject oxygen-rich blood toward the body's tissues. The pulmonary and aortic valves remain open until the end of systole, and then snap shut as the next cardiac cycle begins.

Systole is initiated during the cardiac cycle by the depolarization of specialized cardiac muscle fibers in the upper right wall of the right atrium; this collection of specialized cardiac muscle fibers is called the SA node. The depolarization of the SA node evokes a wave of electrical activity that quickly spreads through the walls of both atria, causing the cardiac muscle fibers in the atrial walls to contract upon depolarization. The wave of electrical activity then momentarily slows down before quickly spreading through the walls of both ventricles, causing the cardiac muscle fibers in the ventricular walls to contract upon depolarization. By the end of systole, all the cardiac muscle fibers in the walls of the atria and ventricles have repolarized. The pattern of depolarization and repolarization of cardiac muscle fibers during the cardiac cycle can be examined by an electrocardiogram (an ECG).

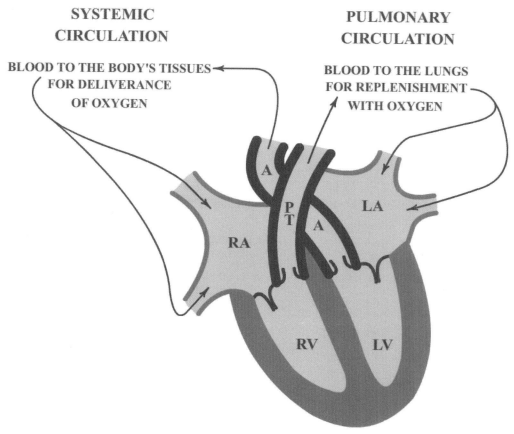

Fig. 5-5: The pulmonary and systemic circulations.

During each cardiac cycle, the right ventricle ejects oxygen-poor blood to the lungs, and the left atrium receives oxygen-rich blood from the lungs (Fig. 5-5). The heart thus sustains a circulation of blood flow between itself and the lungs that serves to replenish the blood's oxygen supply. This circulation of blood flow is called the pulmonary circulation.

During each cardiac cycle, the left ventricle ejects oxygen-rich blood to all the body's tissues, and the right atrium receives oxygen-poor blood from the body's tissues (Fig. 5-5). The heart thus sustains a circulation of blood flow between itself and the body's tissues that serves to deliver oxygen and nutrients to and remove metabolic waste products from all the body's tissues. This circulation of blood flow is called the systemic circulation.

Any irregularity that diminishes blood flow into the atria and ventricles during diastole or the ejection of blood from the ventricles during systole has the potential of producing dyspnea. This is because cardiac dysfunction has the potential of altering blood pressures within the pulmonary circulation and/or blood flow through the pulmonary circulation to the extent that these alterations diminish, through different pathophysiological mechanisms, the lungs' capacity to provide for sufficient exchange of gases between the air breathed into the lungs and the blood pumped through the pulmonary circulation circuit.

We can now examine each of the three categories of cardiac dysfunction that can lead to dyspnea, beginning with pericardial effusion. In the middle of the chest, an inelastic, fibrous sac called the pericardial sac completely encloses the heart. The closed space within the pericardial sac that surrounds the heart is called the pericardial cavity. The inner lining of the pericardial sac secretes a fluid called pericardial fluid that completely fills the pericardial cavity. If the volume of the fluid within the pericardial cavity becomes excessive as a result of infection or injury (a process called pericardial effusion), the subsequent increase in pericardial fluid pressure on the outer surfaces of the heart restricts blood flow into the left and right atria during diastole. The subsequent diminishment of blood flow through the heart's chambers produces dyspnea.

If a third-year or fourth-year medical student were using the diagnostic scheme for dyspnea displayed in Fig. 5-1 in the analysis of a patient, the student would consider the likelihood of cardiac tamponade (the clinical name for severe pericardial effusion) if, in addition to dyspnea, the patient was hypotensive (had markedly low blood pressure) and exhibited distended neck veins because of pooling of blood in the neck veins.

The heart consists of its cardiac muscle fibers and valvular tissue. When a person has a heart attack due to coronary artery disease, some of the cardiac muscle fibers may be at risk of dying due to loss of their own blood supply [coronary arteries are the arteries that supply oxygen-rich blood to the heart itself; coronary artery disease is the disease in which atherosclerotic plaques form on the inner surface of the coronary arteries to the extent that they significantly interfere with coronary artery blood flow]. If the extent of the cardiac muscle fiber death is significant, myocardial dysfunction ensues because the walls of the heart's ventricles cannot move normally. Significant myocardial dysfunction may also occur as a result of alteration of the pattern by which electrical activity spreads throughout the walls of the atria and ventricles during the cardiac cycle. If ventricular pumping activity becomes compromised to the extent that it significantly reduces blood flow through the heart, dyspnea ensues. A third-year or fourth-year medical student would examine an ECG of a patient's heart for evidence of a diagnosis of myocardial dysfunction based on either mechanical or electrical issues.

Each of the heart's four valves is structured to prevent retrograde (that is, backward) blood flow when the valve is closed. Each valve is also structured to facilitate blood flow within the heart or out from the heart when the valve is open. If disease or injury affects the functioning of any of the heart's valves to the extent that it markedly reduces blood flow through the heart's chambers, dyspnea may occur. A third-year or fourth-year medical student would consider the likelihood of valvular dysfunction if, in addition to dyspnea, certain characteristic murmurs were heard during auscultation of the patient's heart sounds. Under normal conditions, only two heart sounds are heard during the cardiac cycle. The first heart sound, called S_1, occurs as a result of the near-simultaneous closure of the mitral and tricuspid valves (the mitral valve is the first of the two valves to close). The second heart sound, S_2, occurs as a result of the near-simultaneous closure of the aortic and pulmonary valves (the aortic valve is the first of the two valves to close). Murmurs are characteristic of turbulent blood flow across an abnormal valve.

You should now begin to appreciate how the diagnostic scheme for dyspnea displayed in Fig. 5-1 could significantly augment your evaluation of a patient who presents with dyspnea as a major complaint. If, upon completing your history and physical exam of the patient, you found evidence of possible cardiac dysfunction but no evidence of pulmonary dysfunction, you would next sequentially consider each major category of cardiac dysfunction. For each major category of cardiac dysfunction, you would compare and contrast the signs and symptoms of the patient's condition with the signs and symptoms that characterize that major category. This is the basic nature of scheme-inductive reasoning. Upon selecting a patient's chief medical problem, that is, his or her clinical presentation, you proceed from possible major categories of dysfunction to progressively smaller and smaller categories of dysfunction to hone in on the most likely diagnosis. At the end of each branch point in the scheme, you compare and contrast the patient's findings with the hallmark characteristics of the dysfunctional category and decide whether or not there is a sufficient match to justify selection of the category. This is how Coderre et al. have described scheme-inductive reasoning:

> "This scheme-inductive process differs from the usual inductive process (reasoning from the clinical data to a diagnosis) in one important manner. It is not simply forward reasoning, 'as reasoning with a single diagnosis in mind'. Decisions are explicitly at the forks in the road or branching of the tree. The organizational structure, or 'scheme' proceeds from alternative causal groups, through 'crucial tests,' to exclusion of some alternative groupings and adoption of what is left. These tests may be based on an evaluation of symptoms, signs, or results of investigations, singly or in any combination."[5-2]

We can now proceed to examine how dysfunction of the mechanics of respiration or the lungs' structural components can produce dyspnea. To do this, we need to describe briefly the gross anatomy of the lungs and the mechanisms by which the lungs are expanded and retracted during breathing.

The total aggregate of airways in a lung is known as its bronchial tree. There are two basic types of airways in the bronchial tree: conduction airways and respiratory airways. The conduction airways are the largest airways of the bronchial tree; they serve only as conduits for the mass flow of air between the trachea and the respiratory airways. The respiratory airways are the smallest airways of the bronchial tree; they provide diffusional exchange of oxygen and carbon dioxide between (a) the air breathed into the lung and (b) the blood in the pulmonary circulation.

The expression 'mechanics of respiration' refers to the structures and forces responsible for breathing, or respiration. Respiration consists of two phases: inspiration, during which air flows into the lungs' airways, and expiration, during which air flows out from the lungs' airways. Air flows into the lungs' airways when the lungs are expanded, and then flows out when the lungs retract. When a lung is expanded, the total volume of its airways increases, and thus the average air pressure within its airways decreases. When this average airway pressure becomes less than atmospheric pressure, air flows into the lung's airways. When the lung subsequently retracts, the average airway pressure increases as the total volume of its airways decreases. When the average airway pressure is greater than that of atmospheric pressure, air flows out from the lung's airways.

The lungs are expanded during inspiration as a consequence of the rib cage moving outward and the diaphragm moving downward (the diaphragm is a thin muscle that separates the chest from the abdomen) (Fig. 5-6). In other words, the lungs cannot by themselves expand their volume; their volume increases during inspiration simply because their outer surfaces follow the outward movement of the rib cage and the downward movement of the diaphragm. However, during expiration, there are both internal and external forces that retract the lungs. During expiration, the lungs retract, in part, as a consequence of the rib cage moving inward and the diaphragm moving upward. The lungs also retract during expiration because of internal retractive forces exerted by lung tissues that were stretched during inspiration. Any disease or injury that weakens the forces that either expand or retract the lungs will reduce the volume of air taken into and then expelled from the lungs during each breath, and thus produce dyspnea.

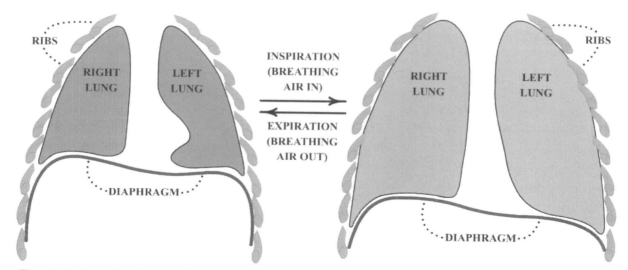

Fig. 5-6: Inspiration and expiration. As the diaphragm descends and the ribs move outward during inspiration, air flows into the lungs' airways. As the diaphragm ascends and the ribs move inward during expiration, air flows out from the lungs' airways.

The walls of the respiratory airways are significantly stretched during inspiration, and it is these stretched walls that provide approximately two-thirds of the internal retractive forces when the lungs retract during expiration. Any disease or injury that narrows the conducting airways may reduce air flow into and out from the lungs to the extent that dyspnea occurs. Similarly, any disease or injury that markedly diminishes either the internal retractive forces of the respiratory airways during expiration or the capacity of the respiratory airways to provide for gaseous exchange will result in dyspnea.

If a third-year or fourth-year medical student were using the diagnostic scheme for dyspnea displayed in Fig. 5-1 in the analysis of a patient, the student would consider a diagnosis of dysfunctional mechanics of respiration if, for example, the student found diminished descent of the patient's diaphragm during inspiration. Disease of the conducting airways would be considered if, for example, the patient exhibited the hallmark characteristics of asthma: episodes of wheezing which the patient describes as periods in which he/she can breathe air into the lungs but has great difficulty in expelling air from the lungs. Disease of the respiratory airways would be considered if, for example, the student found evidence during the physical exam of respiratory airways filled with fluid (such evidence would include abnormal breath and percussion sounds over lung regions densely populated with respiratory airways).

There are three advantages to using scheme-inductive reasoning in examining real or fictional patients during your years in medical school. First, as you have learned from the diagnostic scheme for dyspnea, schemes identify the most likely categories of diseases or injuries that may produce a particular sign, symptom, or abnormal lab test result. If the problem representation of a patient you have examined has not activated recall of an appropriate illness script, selecting the patient's most prominent abnormal finding as the patient's clinical presentation provides at least some degree of order to your diagnostic reasoning if you know one or more diagnostic schemes for that particular clinical presentation. Scheme-inductive reasoning has been shown to improve diagnostic accuracy by medical students during their last year in medical school.[5-2, 5-3] Second, scheme-inductive reasoning focuses on the pathophysiological mechanism of a disease or injury that is responsible for a specific sign, symptom, or abnormal lab test result. Scheme-inductive reasoning thus promotes both the learning and review of the basic medical sciences in relation to the clinical findings of patients. Third and finally, even experienced physicians resort to scheme-inductive reasoning when their knowledge of illness scripts and instance scripts does not adequately account for a patient's health problems.

REFERENCES

5-1. Mandin H, Harasym P, Eagle C, and M Watanabe. Developing A 'Clinical Presentation' Curriculum at the University of Calgary. Academic Medicine (1995) 70:186–193. p. 188.

5-2. Coderre S, Mandin H, Harasym PH, and GH Fick. Diagnostic Reasoning Strategies and Diagnostic Success. Medical Education (2003) 37:695–703. p. 696.

5-3. Coderre S, Jenkins D, and K McLaughlin. Qualitative Differences in Knowledge Structure Are Associated with Diagnostic Performance in Medical Students. Advances in Health Sciences Education: Theory & Practice. (2009) 14:677-684.

Chapter 6

A COURSE ON THE FOUNDATIONS OF DIAGNOSTIC REASONING

In Chapter 1, we began our examination of medical school curricula by discussing the profound impact that Abraham Flexner's 1910 report had on medical education in the United States throughout the 20th Century and continues to have even now into the second decade of the 21st Century. Even before the advent of Knowles' theory of adult learning and the development of contemporary theories of cognitive psychology, Flexner foresaw that basic medical science knowledge should be learned in medical school in relation to the clinical findings of patients. Flexner also recognized that this goal requires more clinical exposure and experience than is currently provided to medical students during their first 18 to 24 months in most medical schools today. The result has been that although medical students in the United States receive superlative basic medical science instruction by Ph.D.s, the cognitive structures in which medical students store this knowledge are difficult to access when the students begin examining real patients in their clinical clerkships. Medical students thus graduate with less than potentially optimal clinical skills, in particular, diagnostic skills.

Charlin et al. have discussed the general parameters by which this fault in current medical school curricula may be addressed:

"The acquisition of diagnosis scripts could be undertaken at the very beginning of medical curricula, and there is a trend in contemporary method of instruction to early exposure to authentic professional tasks; therefore, the desirability of waiting until clerkship to begin the development of scripts adapted to diagnosis tasks is questionable. Early exposure can help students to develop scripts very early and help them to incorporate biomedical and clinical knowledge that they would acquire subsequently within their scripts, if appropriate care is taken about integration of this knowledge. This is in accordance with principles of situated learning. In contrast to such a strategy is the more traditional conception that the construction of biomedical knowledge is a critical foundation phase of medical training and that an early construction of diagnosis scripts would threaten the construction of a strong base of biomedical knowledge.

Whether scripts are built early or later in curricula, their acquisition and refinement cannot be left entirely to the variability of clinical exposure. Knowing that elaborated and organized knowledge is the key to clinical expertise, clinical teachers should explicitly assist students in the construction of efficient and well-structured knowledge bases. Such a knowledge base allows students to give meaning to clinical situations, to guide their clinical inquiry, to interpret clinical information in order to reinforce their hypotheses or weaken them, to activate new ones because entertained ones are not fitted to the situation, and to decide when they have enough data to close the diagnostic process. Educational methods adapted to the requirements of clinical settings have been described.[6-1, 6-2] They follow a series of principles established from cognitive psychology [6-3]: (1) learners actively engage in the educational activity (scripts cannot be transmitted directly from teachers' mind to students' minds; they have to be constructed by each learner); (2) new information is articulated on students' prior knowledge (this implies the activation of prior knowledge); (3) intermediate stages of clinical reasoning are made explicit; (4) students are asked to use their clinical knowledge to assess incoming clinical information and, in so doing, to reinforce or reject entertained hypotheses; and (5) acquired knowledge is validated through its use with peers and teachers."[6-4]

This chapter and the following chapter discuss a relatively modest measure by which a medical school could promote the learning of the basic medical sciences in relation to the clinical findings of patients: Begin medical school with a course titled the Foundations of Diagnostic Reasoning. The course would begin with a straightforward explanation by a clinical instructor of how an experienced physician, while taking a history and performing physical exam procedures on a patient, uses semantic qualifiers, a problem representation, illness scripts, instance scripts and, in some instances, scheme-inductive reasoning, to arrive at a diagnosis of a patient's condition. Such an introduction would last no more than 2 or 3 days.

Then, for 4 to 8 weeks, 2 or 3 cases are presented to the students each week. For each case, the students either watch the history and physical exam of a patient (either real or standardized; either in life or in media) or read a record of a patient's history and physical exam findings before working in teams first to identify the semantic qualifiers of the findings and then to construct a problem representation of the patient. Upon completion of the problem representations by all the student teams, all the problem representations are collected and distributed to all the student teams for class discussion and selection of the team that constructed the best problem representation. A clinical instructor then presents his/her problem representation and facilitates a class discussion of how the clinical instructor's problem representation compares and contrasts with the selection of the class' best problem representation. Next, basic science and clinical instructors facilitate 2 to 3 hour-long sessions for each of 1 to 3 days during which the student teams use digital and book sources to study basic and clinical science material and propose possible diagnoses. Upon identification of possible diagnoses, basic science and clinical instructors facilitate class discussion of the case and provide a general explanation of the disease or injury and the problems associated with its diagnosis. Finally, basic science and clinical instructors facilitate class discussion of an appropriate, tripartite-structured, illness script of the disease or injury.

Assuming that the students could work through 2 to 3 cases per week, it is reasonable to expect that the students could complete approximately 20 cases if the Foundations of Diagnostic Reasoning course was 8 weeks long. The principal guide for the selection of the 20 cases is that, in the aggregate, they present a broad spectrum of common symptoms and signs. For example, the principal symptoms and signs of the cases could consist of the following symptoms and signs, which have been selected from the Calgary Black Book website and listed here in alphabetical order:

Acute Abdominal Pain
Acute Joint Pain
Amenorrhea
Back Pain
Bleeding/Bruising
Chest Discomfort
Cough
Dysphagia
Dyspnea
Fatigue
Fever and Chills
Hypothermia
Jaundice
Localized Lymphadenopathy
Mood Disorder
Nausea and Vomiting

Peripheral Weakness
Polyuria, Polydipsia, and Polyphagia from Diabetes
Sore Throat
Syncope

Observe that, except for the triad of symptoms characteristic of diabetes, there are not any restrictions as to the choice of disease or injury that is selected to highlight each symptom or sign. Although only common diseases or injuries might be considered appropriate, that choice is as appropriate as any other standard. This is because the principal focus of the case exercises in the Foundations of Diagnostic Reasoning course is, except for diabetes, not the cases themselves but rather the symptoms and signs they highlight. It is expected that as the students work through each case, they will learn the nature of the highlighted symptoms and signs and construct one, two, or even more inductive-reasoning schemes by which they explore the pathophysiological basis of the symptoms and signs. These then are the overall learning objectives of this first course in medical school: Upon completion of the course, a student should be able (1) to explain the general nature of each symptom and sign and (2) to evaluate via one or more inductive-reasoning schemes the pathophysiological basis of the symptom or sign.

Although the criteria for selecting the specific cases in the Foundations of Diagnostic Reasoning course are not a critical feature, the signs and symptoms associated with the disease or injury in each case are a critical feature. Each case should present the most common (that is, the most prototypical) signs and symptoms of the disease or injury when the patient is examined at a specific time after the disease began or the injury occurred. This is because each case enables the students to begin construction of an illness script of the disease or injury, and the problem representation that identifies the illness script should be a prototypical problem representation.

Upon achieving the learning objectives of the Foundations of Diagnostic Reasoning course, each student will have begun his/her medical education by learning the semantic qualifiers that apply to 10 to 20 or more signs and symptoms and participated in 10 to 20 student team-based exercises to craft problem representations rich in semantic qualifiers. They will have developed, again in a student team-based environment, schemes for exploring the pathophysiological basis of 10 to 20 problem representations, learning in the process the general basic medical and clinical science knowledge required to describe the pathophysiological basis of each problem representation. They will have thus begun medical school learning the basic medical sciences as they relate to the clinical findings of patients and developed study habits that will sustain this approach as they proceed through their basic medical science courses during the first 18 to 24 months of medical school.

Upon completion of the Foundations of Diagnostic Reasoning course, the medical school can begin its traditional basic medical science courses, be they discipline-based or integrated. It is not necessary during the first year or two following adoption of the Foundations of Diagnostic Reasoning course that any changes be made to other courses with respect to their order in the curriculum, their learning objectives, their learning strategies, or their faculty. Because the students have begun medical school learning about common clinical findings of patients, it is these common clinical findings to which they can now relate anything they learn in a basic medical science course. They entered medical school knowing that learning how to diagnose disease and injury is really the first order of business in medical school, and in the Foundations of Diagnostic Reasoning course, they acquired through team effort the cognitive armamentarium to learn the basic medical sciences in relation to the clinical findings of patients. In every session of a basic medical science course, be it a lecture, lab, or small group exercise, each student has the ability to recognize the relation of what he/she is learning to a sign or symptom that would appear should the structure or process under consideration be altered by disease or injury. Flexner's words are worth repeating here:

> "Undergraduate instruction [that is, instruction in the basic medical sciences] will be throughout explicitly conscious of its professional end and aim. In no other way can all the sciences belonging to the medical curriculum be thoroughly kneaded. An active apperceptive relation must by established and maintained between laboratory and clinical experience. Such a relation cannot be one-sided; it will not spontaneously set itself up in the last two years if it is deliberately suppressed in the first two. There is no cement like interest, no stimulus like the hint of a coming practical application."

From an operational point of view, the singular advantage of beginning medical school with a Foundations of Diagnostic Reasoning course is that it does not require any initial, significant change in the remainder of the medical school curriculum. The only accommodation that has to be made with respect to basic medical science and clinical clerkship instruction is to accommodate the introduction of a 4 to 8-week long course. The Foundations of Diagnostic Reasoning course will facilitate subsequent basic science instruction by introducing key concepts. For example, if dyspnea is selected as one of the symptoms to be analyzed in the Foundations of Diagnostic Reasoning course, the students will learn the basic cardiac and pulmonary anatomy discussed in the previous chapter and thus be prepared to begin their study of the heart and lungs in their anatomy courses at a more detailed level.

As both basic science and clinical faculty acquire experience with the Foundations of Diagnostic Reasoning course, it is likely that both basic science and clinical faculty will begin consideration of changes in their own programs of instruction not only to better complement the overall learning objectives of the Foundations of Diagnostic Reasoning course but also to increasingly promote learning of the basic medical sciences in relation to the clinical findings of patients.

The following chapter presents 5 representative cases that could be developed for a Foundations of Diagnostic Reasoning course. Each case focuses on one or more signs and symptoms of a common disease or condition. Each case provides an opportunity for beginning first-year medical students to identify semantic qualifiers of the signs and symptoms learned from the history and physical exam of a fictional patient and to prepare a problem representation of the patient's condition that is populated with the identified semantic qualifiers. Each case presents an example of a superior, student team-generated problem representation of the patient's condition. Each case discusses the basic medical and clinical science learning objectives that student teams would be expected to attain as they research the pathophysiological mechanism responsible for the patient's condition and discuss their findings in faculty-facilitated class discussion. The learning objectives are stated in terms of Bloom's taxonomy of the cognitive domain. Finally, each case ends with an illness script of a prototypical presentation of the common disease or condition.

You may recall from the beginning of Chapter 1 that this book has been written for you, a first-year medical student. As you study the cases in the following chapter, observe how the cases are designed to promote adult learning behavior by you. For each case, the role of the basic science and clinical instructors is limited to just composing the history and physical exam findings of a fictional patient and defining the learning objectives of the exercise. By contrast, your role would be to work with a team of fellow students to

(1) define the semantic qualifiers of the patient's signs and symptoms,
(2) compose an appropriate problem representation of the patient's condition,
(3) research basic medical and clinical science information necessary to propose one or more inductive-reasoning schemes for diagnosis of the patient's condition, and finally, after the correct diagnosis has been identified,
(4) explain the pathophysiological mechanism responsible for the patient's problem representation.

Each case is thus designed to help you learn, through both individual and group effort, basic medical and clinical science knowledge in the context of the clinical findings of patients. In so doing, you are storing the basic medical and clinical science knowledge in cognitive structures that are most readily recalled by the clinical findings of patients. And, perhaps most importantly, you are acquiring the confidence and skills to assume an active role in your medical education not only in medical school but also throughout the remainder of your career in medicine.

REFERENCES

6-1. Kassirer JP. Teaching Clinical Medicine by Iterative Hypothesis Testing: Let's Preach What We Practice. New England Journal of Medicine. (1983) 309:921-923.

6-2. Chamberland M, Des Marchais JE, and B Charlin. Carrying PBL Into the Clerkship: A Second Reform in the Sherbrooke Curriculum. Ann Community-Oriented Education. (1992) 5:235-247.

6-3. Tardif J. Pour un Enseignement Strategique: l'Apport de la Psychologie Cognitive. Montreal, Quebec, Canada: Les Editions Logiques. 1992.

6-4. Charlin B, Tardif J, and H Boshuizen. Scripts and Medical Knowledge: Theory and Applications for Clinical Reasoning Instruction and Research. Academic Medicine (2000) 75:182-190. p. 188.

Chapter 7

REPRESENTATIVE CASES OF A
FOUNDATIONS OF DIAGNOSTIC REASONING COURSE

CASE 1

A 65 year-old woman has made an appointment with her primary care physician to seek treatment for weakness in her right hand. The following is a transcript of the history taken by the physician and a summary of the physical exam findings:

How are you doing Mrs. Thompson?
- Well, doctor, my right hand is weak. It's become so weak that I have trouble holding a pencil or even holding cards when I play bridge with my friends.

How long has your hand been weak?
- I don't know exactly. It didn't become weak all at once. I'd say that it started about 3 or 4 months ago, but it's become really worse during the last month. I even lost my grip on a cup of hot tea yesterday morning.

Do you feel weakness in any other part of your right arm?
- No, I don't think so. It's just my hand that's weak.

Have you noticed any other problems with your right hand?
- Yes, I've also lost some feeling in my right hand.

Where exactly in your right hand have you lost feeling?
- Right here [the patient uses the index finger of her left hand to point to the palmar surfaces of the thumb, index finger, and middle finger of her right hand] (Fig. 7-1).

How long have you had less feeling in your thumb and fingers?
- Oh, about as long if not longer than my hand has been weak. Like the weakness, it's been getting worse during the last month.

Is there an injury you suffered that you think may be related to your hand problems?
- No, not that I can think of.

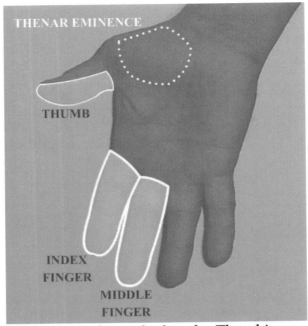

Fig. 7-1: Anterior (palmar) view of a right hand. The skin areas of the thumb, index finger, and middle finger that are shaded white are the skin areas in which the patient has lost feeling. The region of the palm encircled by a dotted white line is the thenar eminence region.

Do you have any weakness or loss of feeling in your left hand?
- No.

Have you had any problems getting out of bed in the morning or rising from a chair?
- No, nothing other than the usual aches and pains.

Have you had any problems standing or walking?
- No.

Is there any other problem you've noticed?
- No.

I recall that you fractured your forearm bone near your right wrist a little over a year ago. I see in my notes from the orthopedist who treated you that the fracture healed well. Has that fracture bothered you at any time?
- No, I don't think so. Could that fracture be the cause of my right hand problems?

I don't know, let's see what I find when I examine your hand. By the way, are you still taking your medications to lower your blood pressure and the cholesterol in your blood?

- Yes.

Physical Exam Findings: Vital signs are normal. System exams are normal except for a diminished thenar eminence, grade 3 strength for opposition, abduction, and flexion of the right thumb, and hypalgesia to pin pricks and hypesthesia to a fine wisp of cotton on the volar surfaces of the thumb and the index and middle fingers of the right hand.

Before turning the page, try to write 1 or 2 sentences with semantic qualifiers that succinctly describe the patient's condition.

The following statement is a superior, student team-generated problem representation of the patient: The patient is a 65 year-old female with insidious onset of grade 3 strength of opposition, abduction, and flexion of the right thumb and hypalgesia and hypesthesia of the volar surfaces of the right thumb, index finger, and middle finger. The prominence of the thenar eminence in the right hand is diminished.

Note the seven semantic qualifiers that populate the patient's problem representation:
(1) The patient's motor and sensory deficits both appeared insidiously; that is, they did not appear abruptly, but rather developed so slowly that the exact time when they began is difficult for the patient to judge.
(2) The motor and sensory deficits appeared almost concurrently.
(3) The motor deficits are limited to opposition, abduction and flexion of the thumb.
(4) Opposition, abduction and flexion of the thumb each exhibit grade 3 muscle strength.
(5) The sensory deficits are confined to only the volar surfaces of the thumb, index finger, and middle finger.
(6) The sensory deficits include both hypalgesia and hypesthesia.
(7) The prominence of the thenar eminence is diminished.

As student teams research the pathophysiological mechanism of the patient's condition and discuss their findings in faculty-facilitated class discussion, it is anticipated that the students would achieve the following basic medical and clinical science learning objectives:

1: A student should be able to recall the clinical names of the digits of the hand.
In the hand, there are 5 digits, and they consist of the four fingers plus the thumb. Each digit can be identified in clinical notes by either one of two equivalent names:
1st Digit – Thumb
2nd Digit – Index Finger
3rd Digit – Middle Finger
4th Digit – Ring Finger
5th Digit – Little Finger
Note, in particular, that the thumb is a digit but should never be called a finger.

2: A student should be able to describe a grading scale for limb muscle strength.
Many examiners assign limb muscle strength in terms of six grades:
Grade 5 represents full and normal strength.
Grade 4 represents strength below normal but great enough to move a limb part against appreciable resistance.
Grade 3 represents strength sufficient to move a limb part against the force of gravity but not great enough to move the limb part against resistance imposed by the examiner.

Grade 2 strength represents strength just sufficient to move a limb part in the absence of the influence of gravity.

Grade 1 represents very severe weakness.

Grade 0 represents complete paralysis.

3: A student should be able to define the following underlined terms and expressions:

The term insidious refers to an event that occurs in a gradual, subtle way.

Opposition of the thumb is the movement in which the tip of the thumb is brought into contact with the tip of any of the fingers.

Abduction of the thumb is the movement in which the thumb is moved forward, or anteriorly, away from the palm of the hand.

Flexion of the thumb is the movement in which the thumb is moved over the surface of the palm toward the medial edge of the palm.

The term hypalgesia refers to decreased sensitivity to painful stimuli.

The term hypesthesia refers to diminished capacity for physical sensation.

The term volar refers to the surfaces of the forearm and hand that are located on the same side as the palm of the hand.

The thenar eminence is the mound of palmar soft tissue at the base of the thumb.

4: A student should be able to recognize that motor and/or sensory deficits in one or more limbs requires consideration of pathophysiological mechanisms/injuries that occurred in not only just the affected limbs themselves but also the brain or spinal cord.

5: A student should be able to explain the prominence of the thenar eminence in the palm of the hand.

The prominence of the thenar eminence is due to the presence of three relatively short muscles in this region of the palm of the hand. The three muscles (opponens pollicis, abductor pollicis brevis, and flexor pollicis brevis) are called the muscles of the thenar eminence, and they all can move the thumb. Opponens pollicis is the only muscle that enables the thumb to be moved so that its tip can touch the tips of the fingers. Abductor pollicis brevis, is, as its name suggests, an abductor of the thumb. Flexor pollicis brevis, as its name suggests, is a flexor of the thumb.

6: A student should be able to describe the basic gross anatomy of the carpal tunnel and its contents.

In the wrist, there is a tunnel-like space called the carpal tunnel that has a bony floor, bony walls, and a thick, inelastic connective tissue roof (Fig. 7-2). The bones of the wrist, the carpals, form the floor and walls of the carpal tunnel, and the thick, inelastic connective tissue roof is called the flexor retinaculum. One of the 5 most prominent nerves of the upper limb, the median nerve, passes through the carpal tunnel as it extends from the forearm into the palm of the hand. The tendons for three forearm muscles also pass through the carpal tunnel as they extend from the forearm into the palm of the hand.

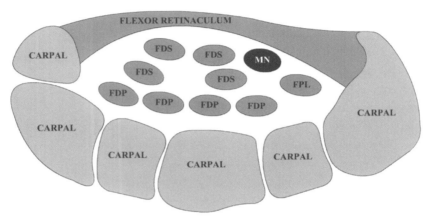

Fig. 7-2: A cross-sectional view of the carpal tunnel in the right wrist as viewed from the forearm. The carpal tunnel transmits the median nerve (MN) and the tendons of three forearm muscles [the four tendons of flexor digitorum superficialis (FDS), the four tendons of flexor digitorum profundus (FDP), and the single tendon of flexor pollicus longus (FPL)]. FDS and FDP each provide a tendon for each of the four fingers, and FPL provides a tendon for the thumb.

7: A student should be able to describe the basic nature of the motor and sensory innervation provided by the median nerve fibers that pass through the carpal tunnel.

Upon entering the palm of the hand, the median nerve provides cutaneous (that is, skin) sensory nerve fibers for the volar surfaces of the thumb, index finger and middle finger and motor nerve fibers for five hand muscles, three of which are the muscles of the thenar eminence.

8: A student should be able to describe the pathophysiological mechanism of the carpal tunnel syndrome.

Any injury or process that increases pressure within the carpal tunnel has the potential of injuring and even ultimately causing the death of both the sensory and motor nerve fibers in the median nerve that pass through the carpal tunnel. This is the pathophysiological mechanism responsible for the signs and symptoms of carpal tunnel syndrome.

9: A student should be able to explain why a primary care physician would recognize that the most likely diagnosis of this case is carpal tunnel syndrome.

The patient's motor and sensory deficits are limited to just those aspects of the motor and sensory innervation of the hand that is provided by the median nerve fibers that extend through the carpal tunnel. In this case, sufficient motor nerve fibers to the muscles of the thenar eminence have been damaged to weaken the opposition, abduction, and flexion movements of the thumb. This partial denervation of the muscles of the thenar eminence has resulted in their atrophy and thus diminishment of the prominence of the thenar eminence. Sufficient cutaneous sensory nerve fibers have also been damaged to account for the patient's loss of feeling on the volar surfaces of her right hand's thumb, index finger, and middle finger. These motor and sensory deficits comprise the prototypical presentation of a severe instance of the condition called the carpal tunnel syndrome.

10: A student should be able to recall an illness script for carpal tunnel syndrome similar to the illness script presented on the following page.

One of the most common causes of carpal tunnel syndrome is repetitive motion of the hand at the wrist. Such repetitive motion occurs among individuals whose occupation involves working on a computer keyboard for several hours every working day or working on an assembly line that requires repetitive hand motions. Another predisposing condition for carpal tunnel syndrome is a Colles' fracture. A Colles' fracture is a fracture of the distal end (the end near the wrist) of the radius. The following website has a drawing of a Colles' fracture: http://orthoinfo.aaos.org/topic.cfm?topic=a00412. Colles' fractures are a relatively common injury among elderly individuals. The distal end of the radius is a common site for osteoporosis among older individuals, and the subsequent loss of bone mass at the distal end of the radius increases the likelihood of a facture occurring if the individual falls down on an outstretched hand.

ILLNESS SCRIPT FOR
CARPAL TUNNEL SYNDROME

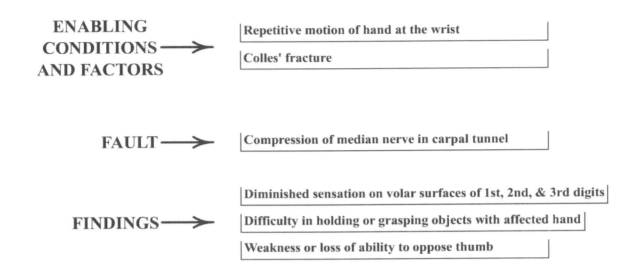

ENABLING CONDITIONS AND FACTORS ⟶
| Repetitive motion of hand at the wrist |
| Colles' fracture |

FAULT ⟶
| Compression of median nerve in carpal tunnel |

FINDINGS ⟶
| Diminished sensation on volar surfaces of 1st, 2nd, & 3rd digits |
| Difficulty in holding or grasping objects with affected hand |
| Weakness or loss of ability to oppose thumb |

In the clinical presentation curriculum developed by the University of Calgary Faculty of Medicine, a clinical representation of peripheral weakness with sensory deficits represents a neurological disorder. The scheme-inductive process for resolving the cause of this particular case of peripheral weakness with sensory deficits ultimately focuses on whether disease or injury of (a) an individual spinal nerve, (b) an individual peripheral nerve, or (c) multiple peripheral nerves best accounts for the patient's signs and symptoms.

CASE 2

A 15 year-old girl has made an appointment with her pediatrician to seek evaluation of recent weight loss. The following is a transcript of the history taken by the physician and a summary of the physical exam findings:

I see here from the nurse's notes that you are concerned about a recent loss in your weight. How much weight have you lost?

- About eight pounds.

When did you notice that you were starting to lose weight?

- Oh, maybe about 2 or 3 weeks ago.

Did you start a diet in order to try to lose weight?

- No. In fact, if anything, I've started eating more, even more than my brother. That's why my mother is worried that I'm losing weight.

As I recall, you brother is about a year younger than you. Is that right?

- Yea.

Have you changed the kinds of food you normally eat?

- No, not really.

Is there anything else that is bothering you, or that you think may be associated with your weight loss?

- Well, I don't know, but I feel tired a lot, and I'm always thirsty. I'm even drinking more soda than my brother.

How long have you felt tired?

- Oh, it started about 2 weeks ago.

Have you been getting enough sleep?

- Yea, I sleep well.

Have you changed your exercise or sports activities in the last few weeks?

- No.

Have long have you noticed your increased thirst?

- Oh, for about the last 2 weeks.

Do you urinate a lot?

- Yea, now that you mention it.

Physical Exam Findings: Vital signs and system exams are normal.

Before turning the page, try to write 1 or 2 sentences with semantic qualifiers that succinctly describe the patient's condition.

The following statement is a superior, student team-generated problem representation of the patient: The patient is a 15 year-old female who reports recent weight loss of 8 pounds, fatigue, polyphagia, polydipsia, and polyuria.

As student teams research the pathophysiological mechanism of the patient's condition and discuss their findings in faculty-facilitated class discussion, it is anticipated that the students would achieve the following basic medical and clinical science learning objectives:

1: A student should be able to define the following underlined terms:
    The term polyphagia refers to excessive eating of food.
    The term polydipsia refers to excessive thirst and fluid intake.
    The term polyuria refers to excessive passage of urine.

 2: A student should be able to discuss basic facts about how fuel metabolism is regulated throughout the body, such as
   (a) the blood-borne hormones that exert the greatest roles,
   (b) the cells whose major metabolic fuel pathways exert the greatest roles,
   (c) the chemical nature of the major metabolic fuels in the blood circulation, and
   (d) the chemical nature of the body's major intracellular storage forms of metabolic fuel.
    Fuel metabolism is regulated throughout the body by blood-borne hormones. The hormones that are most important in this respect are insulin, glucagon, and catecholamines. Endocrine cells in the pancreas called β cells are the source of insulin that is secreted into the blood; other endocrine cells in the pancreas called α cells are the source of glucagon that is secreted into the blood. Endocrine cells in the adrenal glands are the source of the two catecholamines (epinephrine and norepinephrine) that are secreted into the blood.
    Insulin, glucagon, and catecholamines regulate the major metabolic fuel pathways in the liver's principal cells (the hepatocytes), the skeletal muscle fibers of the body's skeletal muscles, and the fat cells of the body's fat tissues. This regulation is the basis of the control that the hormones exert on fuel metabolism throughout the body.
    Through their regulation of the major metabolic fuel pathways in these cells, the hormones control the blood levels of glucose and free fatty acids, which are the major metabolic fuels in the blood circulation. In particular, the hormones attempt to maintain a blood glucose concentration of about 90 mg/dl. A minimum blood glucose level needs to be maintained because the cells of the brain are almost completely dependent upon a continuous supply of blood-borne glucose for their energy metabolism.

Through their regulation of the major metabolic fuel pathways in hepatocytes, skeletal muscle fibers, and fat cells, the hormones also control the build-up and breakdown of glycogen and fat, which are the body's intracellular storage forms of metabolic fuel. Glycogen, which is polymerized glucose, is stored in mainly hepatocytes and skeletal muscle fibers. Fat consist of triacylglyerols; triacylglycerols are molecules in which three fatty acid chains are bound covalently to a single glycerol molecule. Fat is stored in fat cells.

3: A student should be able to describe the basic effects of insulin versus glucagon and catecholamines on
  (a) the major metabolic fuels in the blood circulation and
  (b) the major intracellular storage forms of metabolic fuel.
   In regulating fuel metabolism, insulin acts to lower the levels of glucose and free fatty acids in the blood and build up glycogen and fat deposits. Glucagon and the catecholamines, on the other hand, stimulate the breakdown of glycogen and fat deposits to raise the levels of glucose and free fatty acids in the blood. Glucagon increases the blood glucose level by also stimulating the liver to synthesize glucose for the blood. The actions of glucagon and the catecholamines on fuel metabolism are thus counter-regulatory to insulin's actions.

4: A student should be able to define the two basic states of fuel metabolism when a person is at rest.
   There are two basic states of fuel metabolism when a person is at rest: the anabolic state and the catabolic state. The anabolic state is characteristic of fuel metabolism when ingested foodstuffs are being digested and absorbed into the blood circulation. The body switches to the catabolic state when the foodstuffs from the most recent meal have been digested and absorbed completely from the small intestine. Upon ingestion of the next meal, the body switches back again to the anabolic state during the postprandial period, which is the 1 to 2 hour period following ingestion of the meal.

5: A student should be able to discuss the major metabolic pathways that characterize fuel metabolism when ingested foodstuffs are being digested and absorbed into the blood circulation.

Fig. 7-3 displays the major metabolic pathways among the liver's hepatocytes, skeletal muscle fibers, and fat cells when the body is in the anabolic state. The transition from a catabolic state to an anabolic state occurs basically as a consequence of increased secretion of insulin into the blood circulation by the β cells of the pancreas. When the body is in the anabolic state, insulin controls fuel metabolism. In the anabolic state, foodstuffs are being digested and absorbed by the small intestine. Proteins are digested into amino acids, complex carbohydrates are digested into glucose and other simple sugars, and fats are digested into fatty acids. The amino acids and glucose absorbed by the small intestine pass into a vein called the portal vein, which conveys its blood into the liver. In the liver, the hepatocytes take up much of the amino acids and glucose. The fatty acids absorbed by the small intestine are synthesized in the small intestine into fat, which is then packaged in particles called chylomicrons and conveyed by lymphatic vessels into the blood circulation.

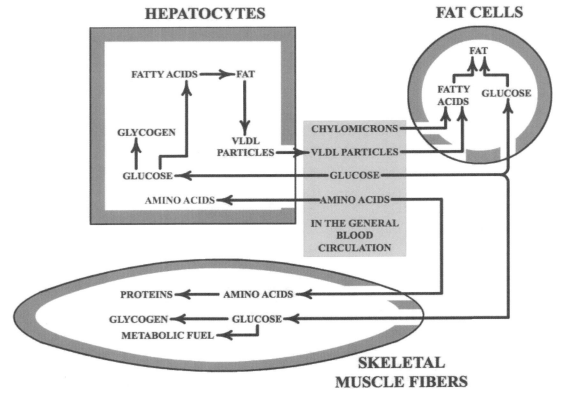

Fig. 7-3: The control of anabolic metabolism by insulin.

In the liver's hepatocytes, some of the absorbed glucose is polymerized into glycogen. Another portion of the glucose is used to synthesize fatty acids, which are then synthesized into fats that are packaged into particles called VLDL particles (VLDL stands for very low density lipoprotein). The VLDL particles are released into the blood circulation.

Observe that when glucose is being acquired from the diet in the anabolic state, the liver lowers the blood glucose level by absorbing glucose from the blood circulation and either polymerizing it into intrahepatic glycogen or converting it into fatty acids which are stored as fat in fat cells.

As chylomicrons and VLDL particles enter the blood capillary beds of fat tissues when the body is in the anabolic state, an insulin-stimulated lipoprotein lipase in the blood capillary beds breaks down the fat in the chylomicrons and VLDL particles into fatty acids, which then enter the fat cells and are re-incorporated into fat. In the anabolic state, fat cells act to store as fat some of the glucose and fatty acids that were acquired from the last meal.

In the anabolic state, skeletal muscle fibers absorb glucose from the blood circulation and partly store it in the form of glycogen, with the remainder being used as metabolic fuel. The skeletal muscle fibers also absorb amino acids from the blood circulation to synthesize intracellular proteins.

6: A student should be able to discuss the major metabolic pathways that characterize fuel metabolism in the liver's hepatocytes, skeletal muscle fibers, and fat cells following an overnight fast.

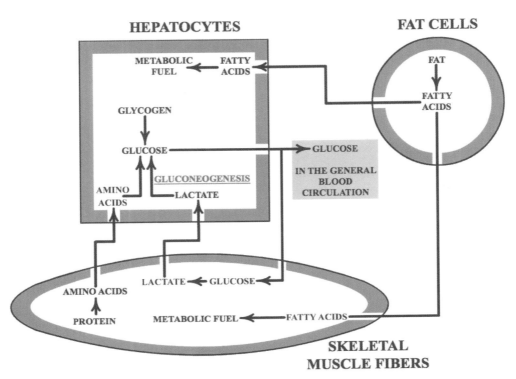

Fig. 7-4: The control of catabolic metabolism by glucagon and the catecholamines.

Following an overnight fast, the body is in the catabolic state, and glucagon and the catecholamines control fuel metabolism (Fig. 7-4). In the absence of glucose being acquired from the diet, the liver produces glucose at a rate equal to that of its consumption by the cells and tissues of the body. In other words, glucose production by the liver becomes largely responsible for maintaining the normal blood glucose level. To sustain this rate of glucose production, the liver's hepatocytes produce glucose via two pathways: glycogen breakdown and gluconeogenesis. Gluconeogenesis is a pathway by which glucose is synthesized from amino acids and lactate. The amino acids and lactate are acquired from reactions in skeletal muscle fibers. The liver and skeletal muscles continuously engage in a cyclical process in which the liver produces glucose for its energy-producing breakdown into lactate in skeletal muscle fibers as the skeletal muscle fibers produce lactate for gluconeogenesis in the liver. This cyclical process is called the Cori cycle.

In the catabolic state, fat cells break down their fat deposits, producing in the process free fatty acids that are used as metabolic fuel by most of the body's tissues.

7: A student should be able to distinguish between the pathophysiological mechanisms of Type 1 versus Type 2 diabetes.

Diabetes is the principal disorder of fuel metabolism. Diabetes mellitus is the disease that results when there is a significant decrease in insulin action. There are two main types of diabetes: Type 1, or insulin-dependent, diabetes mellitus and Type 2, or insulin-independent diabetes mellitus. Whereas persons with Type 1 diabetes absolutely cannot live without insulin administration, persons with Type 2 diabetes can.

Persons with Type 1 diabetes suffer from autoimmune destruction of the β cells in the pancreas and thus eventually suffer from extremely low blood insulin levels. This marked decrease in the blood insulin level accounts for the decrease in insulin action in persons with Type 1 diabetes.

By contrast, persons with Type 2 diabetes have functional β cells in the pancreas and blood insulin levels that may be in the normal concentration range. However, they suffer from two defects: First, regulation of insulin secretion is abnormal; the β cells do not secrete insulin in amounts sufficient to appropriately control the blood glucose level. Second, insulin exerts less than normal effects on the liver, skeletal muscles, and fat tissues. The inadequate insulin secretion by β cells and the resistance of the liver, skeletal muscles, and fat tissues to respond adequately to insulin together account for the decrease in insulin action in persons with Type 2 diabetes.

In persons with either untreated Type 1 or untreated Type 2 diabetes, the decrease in insulin action leads ultimately to hyperglycemia (an abnormally high blood glucose level) and hypertriglyceridemia (abnormally high concentrations of fat in the blood circulation).

The focus in this case is on only Type 1 diabetes. This is because when a child or an adolescent is afflicted with diabetes, Type 1 diabetes is more common.

<u>8</u>: A student should be able to discuss the major metabolic pathways that characterize fuel metabolism in the liver's hepatocytes, skeletal muscle fibers, and fat cells when a person is suffering from untreated Type 1 diabetes.

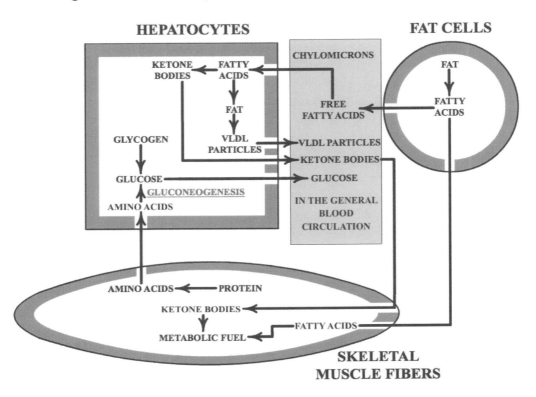

Fig. 7-5: The extreme form of catabolic metabolism with untreated Type 1 diabetes.

In healthy persons, the lowest blood insulin levels occur during fasting periods. The basal level of insulin in the blood during these fasting periods exerts a restraining effect on the metabolic fuel pathways that glucagon and catecholamines stimulate in the liver, skeletal muscles, and fat tissues. However, in persons with untreated Type 1 diabetes, ultimately there is almost no restraining effect exerted by insulin because of the extremely low blood insulin level. Therefore, in persons with untreated Type 1 diabetes, the body exerts an extreme form of catabolic metabolism (Fig. 7-5). This extreme form of catabolic metabolism occurs not only during fasting periods but also after meals, because the blood insulin level does not significantly increase upon absorption of glucose and amino acids from the small intestine.

The extreme form of catabolic metabolism expressed in person with untreated Type 1 diabetes features accelerated fat breakdown in fat cells, accelerated protein breakdown in skeletal muscle fibers and accelerated glycogen breakdown, gluconeogenesis, ketogenesis (synthesis of ketone bodies from fatty acids), and VLDL production in hepatocytes.

The accelerated glycogen breakdown and gluconeogenesis in the liver and the absence of insulin-stimulated glucose uptake by skeletal muscle fibers and fat cells combine to produce hyperglycemia.

The accelerated fat breakdown in fat cells produces an abundant supply of free fatty acids in the blood circulation. The marked increase in the blood level of free fatty acids produces, by mass effect, a marked increase in fatty acid uptake and utilization by, in particular, skeletal muscle fibers and hepatocytes. Skeletal muscle fibers preferentially use the fatty acids as metabolic fuel. In the hepatocytes, the fatty acids increase, again by mass effect, the production of VLDL particles and ketone bodies. The fatty acid-driven production of VLDL particles by hepatocytes and the absence of insulin-stimulated lipoprotein lipase activity in the blood capillary beds of fat tissues combine to produce hypertriglyceridemia. The fatty acid-driven production of ketone bodies leads to hyperketonemia. It is important to recognize that, in persons with untreated Type I diabetes, the accelerated hepatic ketogenesis is largely a result of the accelerated fat breakdown in the body's fat cells.

9: A student should be able to describe the development of ketoacidosis in a person suffering from untreated Type 1 diabetes.

When the blood insulin level becomes extremely low in persons with untreated Type 1 diabetes, fat breakdown in fat cells becomes virtually unchecked. The unchecked fat breakdown generates unchecked ketogenesis in hepatocytes. The resulting hyperketonemia becomes so great that the blood pH decreases; this is because ketone bodies are organic acids. The lowering of the blood pH that occurs from extreme hyperketonemia is called ketoacidosis. Persons with Type 1 diabetes are said to be ketoacidosis-prone because, in the absence of treatment, the blood insulin level can drop so low that fat breakdown in fat cells (a rate-limiting step for hepatic ketogenesis) becomes virtually unchecked.

10: A student should be able to describe how untreated Type 1 diabetes produces the classical initial symptoms of polyuria, polydipsia and polyphagia.

Polyuria develops as a result of hyperglycemia. The excessive loss of water from the polyuria produces persistent thirst and thus polydipsia. "In diabetes mellitus, glucose utilization is reduced in the cells of the satiety center [in the brain], which therefore signals a glucose deficiency to the feeding center. As a result, hunger is perceived, and food intake increases" [Michael, J and S. Sircar. Fundamentals of Medical Physiology 2010 Thieme. p. 521].

The mechanism by which hyperglycemia produces polyuria relates to how the kidneys regulate the amount of blood glucose that is excreted in urine. The kidneys cleanse the blood of metabolic waste products by first producing an ultrafiltrate of blood plasma (blood plasma is the fluid, cell-free fraction of blood). The concentration of glucose in the ultrafiltrate is the same as that in the blood. The kidneys then recover almost all the nutrients and important ions and most of the water from the ultrafiltrate (leaving behind metabolic waste products). Glucose is among the nutrients recovered from the ultrafiltrate. However, there is a maximum rate at which glucose can be recovered from the ultrafiltrate. When the blood glucose level becomes as great or greater than 16 mM, the kidneys cannot recover all of the glucose in the ultrafiltrate, and the unrecovered glucose is then excreted in the urine. Glycosuria (glucose in the urine) thus occurs when hyperglycemia approaches or exceeds 16 mM.

The glucose in the ultrafiltrate that cannot be recovered exerts an osmotic force that decreases water recovery by the kidneys. This process by which unrecovered glucose in the ultrafiltrate decreases water recovery is called osmotic diuresis. In sum, persons with untreated Type 1 diabetes develop glycosuria when their hyperglycemia exceeds the capacity of the kidneys to recover all the glucose in the ultrafiltrate. The glycosuria produces, in turn, polyuria via osmotic diuresis.

11: A student should be able to recall an illness script for Type 1 diabetes similar to the illness script presented here.

The triad of polyphagia, polydipsia, and polyuria is pathognomonic for diabetes. Observe that both genetic factors and viral infection may contribute to the genesis of Type 1 diabetes. If both of a child's parents have Type 1 diabetes, the child's risk for Type 1 diabetes ranges from 10 to 25% [http://www.diabetes.org/diabetes-basics/genetics-of-diabetes.html]. "Common intestinal infections caused by human enteroviruses (HEVs) are considered major environmental factors predisposing to Type 1 diabetes" [http://www.ncbi.nlm.nih.gov/pubmed/20680525].

ILLNESS SCRIPT FOR
TYPE 1 DIABETES MELLITUS

ENABLING CONDITIONS AND FACTORS ⟶

Genetic factors; 10-25% risk if both parents have Type 1 diabetes
Viral infection (enterovirus)

FAULT ⟶

Autoimmune destruction of beta cells in pancreas

FINDINGS ⟶

Polyuria, polydipsia, and polyphagia
Fatigue
Weight loss

In the clinical presentation curriculum developed by the University of Calgary Faculty of Medicine, a clinical presentation of recent, unexplained weight loss represents a gastrointestinal disorder. The scheme-inductive process for resolving the cause of weight loss focuses first on the general nature of the cause: is the weight loss the result of (a) environmental/social factors, (b) a psychiatric/psychological condition, or (c) somatic disease (a bodily illness)?

CASE 3

A 67 year-old man has made an appointment with his primary care physician to seek treatment for lower back pain. The following is a transcript of the history taken by the physician and a summary of the physical exam findings:

How are you doing Mr. Mullen?
- I've been having pain in my lower back for about 3 months.

Do you have back pain now?
- Yes.

Can you show me or describe to me where you feel pain?
- Back here (the patient places his right hand over the lumbar region of the spine).

How would you describe the pain?
- It just feels like an ache in my back.

If you think back to when the pain started, might it be the result of you twisting your back or accidentally falling down?
- No, nothin' like that. All I know is that the pain started gradually about 3 months ago.

Has the nature of the pain or its location changed at any time during the past 3 months?
- No, not really.

Have you found that the back pain becomes worse if you bend your back in a particular way?
- No.

Have you found that the back pain becomes momentarily worse when you cough, sneeze, or bear down during a bowel movement?
- No.

How about if you try to pick up something that's heavy?
- No.

Have you found anything that relieves the pain?
- Well, if I lie down, the pain seems a bit better, but it's still there.

Is there anything else that is also bothering you?

- No.

Have you had any recent injuries or illnesses?

- No.

Do you have any respiratory problems, such as a cough or shortness of breath?

- Well, I've had a morning cough for about 4 years. I generally cough every morning to clear my lungs.

What generally is the color of the sputum?

- It's yellowish or brownish.

Do you ever cough up blood?

- Oh, once or twice I've seen a speck of blood in the sputum I've coughed up in the morning.

Are you still smoking?

- Yes, I know you've wanted me to stop smoking, but it's really difficult. I still smoke about a pack of cigarettes a day.

Have you had any recent problems with urination?

- Well, I do have trouble starting and stopping. The urine will sometimes dribble out before I can get to the bathroom.

Is it ever painful to urinate?

- No.

Have you found that you have to get up frequently at night to urinate?

- Yes. I go about 3 or 4 times a night. I guess my bladder must be weak because I don't generally pass much urine.

Has there been any recent change in your weight?

- Yes, I've lost about 10 pounds in the last 3 months.

Have you changed your diet in the last few months?

- No, not really.

Are you still taking your high blood pressure and cholesterol medicine?

- Yes.

Physical Exam Findings: BP: 130/80. System exams are normal except for a few expiratory rhonchi throughout both lungs and a hard, irregular painless nodule in the right lateral lobe of the prostate.

Before turning the page, try to write 1 or 2 sentences with semantic qualifiers that succinctly describe the patient's condition.

The following statement is a superior, student team-generated problem representation of the patient: The patient is a 67 year-old male with chronic bronchitis, insidious low back pain of 3 months duration, and recent urgency, dysuria, nocturia, and weight loss of 10 pounds. Digital rectal examination finds a hard, painless prostatic nodule.

As student teams research the pathophysiological mechanism of the patient's condition and discuss their findings in faculty-facilitated class discussion, it is anticipated that the students would achieve the following basic medical and clinical science learning objectives:

1: A student should be able to define the following underlined terms:
   The term bronchitis refers to inflammation of the trachea and the conducting airways of the lungs.
   The term rhonchi refers to snore-like lung sounds.
   The term micturition refers to the discharge of urine.
   The term urgency refers to a sudden desire to urinate.
   The term dysuria refers to difficulty with urination.
   The term nocturia refers to excessive urination at night.
   The expression digital rectal examination (DRE) refers to physical examination of the anal canal and rectum (the two lowest regions of the digestive tract) via a gloved finger.

2: A student should be able to describe the skeletal framework of the lumbosacral region of the spine.
   Lower back pain is pain in the lumbosacral region of the spine. The lumbosacral region of the spine is the region occupied by the 5 lumbar vertebrae and the sacrum (Fig. 7-6). The sacrum is a wedge-shaped bone of the spine that forms during childhood and adolescence from the fusion of 5 sacral vertebrae. On each side of the body, the sacrum is joined to the hip bone by a joint called the sacroiliac joint.

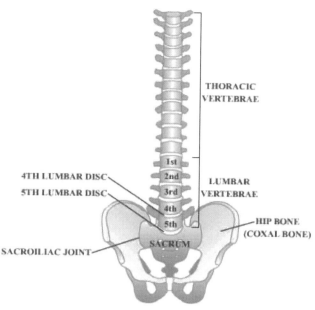

Fig. 7-6: Anterior view of the thoracic vertebrae, lumbar vertebrae, and sacrum of the spine and the paired hip bones.

3: A student should be able to recall that there are two major categories of the etiology (cause) of lower back pain: mechanical versus nonmechanical causes (Fig. 7-7).

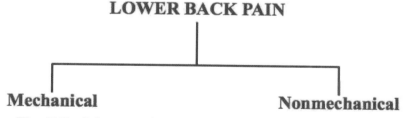

Fig. 7-7: Scheme of major causes of lower back pain.

4: A student should be able to describe the general nature of mechanical causes of lower back pain and recall at least two specific mechanical causes of lower back pain.

Mechanical causes are disorders intrinsic to the spine produced by excessive strain on or degenerative changes in its musculoskeletal framework. Mechanical causes include musculotendinous or ligamentous strains, herniated intervertebral discs, degenerative changes such as spondylosis (stiffening or fixation of the spine's joints as a result of the formation of fibrous or bony structures between joint surfaces) or spondylolysis (the breaking down of a vertebra), and compression fracture of the body of a lumbar vertebra (Fig. 7-8).

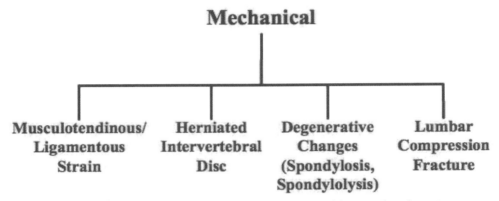

Fig. 7-8: Scheme of mechanical causes of lower back pain.

5: A student should be able to describe the signs and symptoms that suggest lower back pain of mechanical origin.

If a patient reports that spinal movements or activities that change pressure along the length of the spine change either the intensity or location of lower back pain, then it is likely that the lower back pain is of mechanical origin. Activities that change pressure along the length of the spine include coughing, sneezing, bearing down during a bowel movement, and lifting a heavy object.

Radicular pain also suggests lower back pain of mechanical origin. Radicular pain is pain produced by compression and/or inflammation of the roots of one or more spinal nerves. For example, observe that the two lowest intervertebral discs in the spine are the 4th and 5th lumbar discs (each intervertebral disc is named according to the number and name of the vertebra immediately above it) (Fig. 7-6). The 4th and 5th lumbar discs are the most commonly herniated discs in the lumbar region of the spine. When the 4th lumbar disc is herniated, it most commonly compresses the roots of the 5th lumbar nerve (whose abbreviated clinical name is L5). When the 5th lumbar disc is herniated, it most commonly compresses the roots of the first sacral spinal nerve (whose abbreviated clinical name is S1). L5 and S1 are two of the five spinal nerves that contribute nerve fibers to the largest nerve of the human body: the sciatic nerve. The sciatic nerve is one of the three largest nerves that innervates muscles and skin of the lower limb. It extends through the lower limb by descending through the buttock and the back of the thigh. Compression of the roots of either L5 or S1 by a herniated intervertebral disc commonly evokes pain that may radiate (that is, extend) from the buttock into the back of the thigh. Such radiation of pain from the compressed root of a spinal nerve is called radicular pain.

<u>6</u>: A student should be able to explain why, in taking the history of the patient, the physician explored the likelihood of mechanical causes of lower back pain before exploring the likelihood of nonmechanical causes.

The physician initiated the inquiry into the origin and nature of the patient's lower back pain with questions pertaining to mechanical causes because the etiology of lower back pain is most commonly a mechanical cause. Having found no evidence from the patient that the intensity or location of his lower back pain changes with spinal movements or activities that change the pressure along the length of the spine, the physician began his investigation of nonmechanical causes of the lower back pain by asking open-ended questions about the patient's respiratory and urinary systems.

<u>7</u>: A student should be able to explain why the physician explored the likelihood of nonmechanical causes of lower back pain by asking open-ended questions about the patient's respiratory and urinary systems.

The physician recognized that the nonmechanical causes of lower back pain are all conditions that are potentially debilitating or fatal (Fig. 7-9). The debilitating or fatal nature of the nonmechanical causes of lower back pain is emphasized in Fig. 7-9 by the listing of the nonmechanical causes in an order in which the first letters of the first words of the nonmechanical causes all together spell the word "OMINOUS."

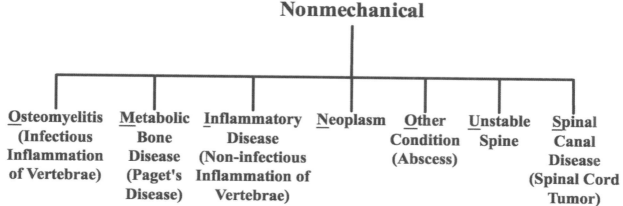

Fig. 7-9: Scheme of nonmechanical causes of lower back pain.

The physician recognized that of the nonmechanical causes of lower back pain, the patient has, in particular, factors that predispose him to neoplasm. The patient's past and present history of cigarette smoking has increased his risk of lung cancer, and his advanced age has increased his risk of prostate cancer. Furthermore, it is common for cancer of the lungs or prostate to metastasize (spread) to the vertebrae of the spine. It is for these reasons that the physician inquired if the patient has any recent pulmonary or urinary problems.

The patient's chronic productive cough (the cough produces sputum) and expiratory rhonchi throughout both lungs are manifestations of chronic bronchitis (chronic inflammation of the lung's conducting airways). The inflammation produces excessive bronchial secretions, and it is the turbulent passage of air through these excessive secretions that generates the rhonchi. These findings neither increase nor decrease the likelihood of lung cancer.

The patient's report of recent problems with urinary retention prompted the physician to consider disease or disorder of the urinary bladder and/or prostate. The neck of the urinary bladder, which is the lowest region of the bladder, gives rise to the urethra (Fig 7-10). The urethra conducts urine from the bladder to the exterior. In a male, the urethra, upon emerging from the neck of the bladder, immediately extends through the prostate (the prostate is a gland which contributes secretions to ejaculate). The segment of the urethra in a male that extends through the prostate is called the prostatic urethra.

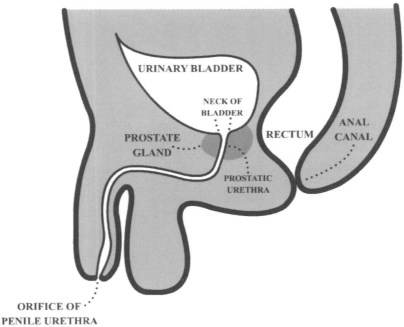

Fig. 7-10: Lateral (side) view of the anatomical relationships of the urinary bladder, prostate gland, rectum and anal canal in a male.

<u>8</u>: A student should be able to describe common causes of urgency, dysuria, and nocturia in an older male.

A finding of urgency, dysuria, and nocturia in a male suggests (a) infectious inflammation of the urinary bladder, prostate, or urethra or (b) altered configuration of the urethrovesical junction, which is the junction between the neck of the urinary bladder and the prostatic urethra (Fig. 7-11).

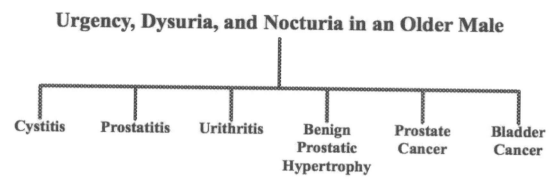

Fig. 7-11: Scheme of causes for urgency, dysuria, and nocturia in an older male.

Cystitis, prostatitis, and urethritis are, respectively, infectious inflammation of the urinary bladder, prostate, and urethra. Pain upon urination suggests urethritis. Benign prostatic hypertrophy is benign enlargement of the prostate, a condition that occurs to some extent in most men after the age of 50. In this case, the finding of a hard, painless prostatic nodule upon rectal examination strongly indicates prostate cancer.

<u>9</u>: A student should be able to explain the pathophysiological mechanism by which prostate cancer can produce urgency, dysuria, and nocturia in a male.

In this case, the enlargement of the malignant nodule in the prostate has distorted the configuration of the urethrovesical junction to the extent that the neck of the bladder can no longer restrict the passage of urine into the urethra. Passage of urine into the urethral segment immediately distal to the neck of the bladder stimulates sensory fibers that provoke an intense urge to urinate. It is through this pathophysiological mechanism that an altered configuration of the urethrovesical junction can cause urgency, nocturia, and difficulty in terminating urine flow at the end of micturition.

10: A student should be able to explain the anatomical findings provided by a digital rectal exam (DRE) in male patients suspected of having prostate disease.

In a male, the urethra, upon emerging from the neck of the bladder, immediately extends through the prostate gland (Fig. 7-10). The prostate gland lies immediately anterior to (in front of) the lowest region of the rectum (the rectum and anal canal are the two lowest segments of the digestive tract). If a gloved finger is inserted through the anal canal and into the lowest region of the rectum in a male, the posterior aspect of the prostate gland can be palpated. Palpation can provide evidence of the size and firmness of the prostate as well as the presence of any irregularities in the contour of the posterior surface of the gland. However, it is important to recognize that digital rectal examination alone cannot differentiate benign prostatic hypertrophy from prostate cancer.

11: A student should be able to explain why prostate cancer commonly metastasizes to the vertebrae of the spine.

When malignant cells begin shedding from the site of a primary prostate tumor, it is common for some of them to enter the veins that drain the prostate gland. These veins communicate directly with a vertebral venous plexus that extends superiorly (upward) along the length of the spine to communicate ultimately with the venous sinuses in the skull (which are called the dural venous sinuses). The dural venous sinuses receive blood that is drained from the brain. In 1940, Oscar Batson conducted studies that proved the continuity of prostatic veins with the vertebral venous plexus and proposed that these venous connections provide a route by which malignant prostate cells can metastasize from the prostate gland to the vertebrae of the spine. [Batson OV. The Function of the Vertebral Veins and Their Role in the Spread of Metastases. Annals of Surgery. (1940) 112:138-149] "Today the vertebral venous plexus is considered part of the cerebrospinal venous system, which is regarded as a unique, large capacitance, valveless plexiform venous network (in which flow is bi-directional) that plays an important role in the regulation of intracranial pressure with changes in posture and in venous outflow from the brain, whereas in disease states, it provides a potential route for the spread of tumor, infection, or emboli." [Nathoo N, Caris EC, Wiener JA, and E Mendel. History of the Vertebral Venous Plexus and the Significant Contributions of Breschet and Batson. Neurosurgery. (2011) 69:1007-1014. p. 1007]

In this case, when malignant prostate cells spread to the lumbar vertebrae of the spine via the vertebral venous plexus, they became established in the parts of the vertebrae bearing hematopoetic (that is, blood-forming) marrow. As the malignant cells proliferated in the marrow, microfractures occurred as a result of the disorganization of bony trabeculae (bony trabeculae are minute beams of bone tissue within the vertebrae). The expanding metastases and the microfractures in the lumbar vertebrae are responsible for the patient's lower back pain.

One further remark is necessary here at the conclusion of this case. Even though metastatic prostate cancer is almost the only plausible diagnosis that can account for the finding of a hard, painless prostatic nodule upon rectal examination of a fictional patient with insidious, unremitting lower back pain, in the real world, radiological studies and lab tests would have to be conducted to verify the diagnosis and also to examine whether the patient may also be suffering from lung cancer or lung metastases.

11: A student should be able to recall an illness script for prostate cancer similar to the illness script presented here. However, it bears repeating that digital rectal examination alone cannot differentiate benign prostatic hypertrophy from prostate cancer.

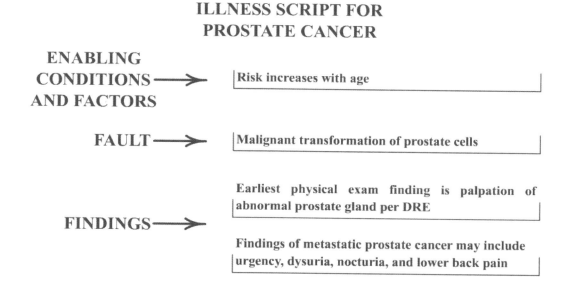

ILLNESS SCRIPT FOR
PROSTATE CANCER

ENABLING CONDITIONS AND FACTORS ⟶ | Risk increases with age |

FAULT ⟶ | Malignant transformation of prostate cells |

FINDINGS ⟶ | Earliest physical exam finding is palpation of abnormal prostate gland per DRE |

| Findings of metastatic prostate cancer may include urgency, dysuria, nocturia, and lower back pain |

In the clinical presentation curriculum developed by the University of Calgary Faculty of Medicine, a clinical presentation of back pain (axial spine pain) represents a neurological disorder. The scheme-inductive process for resolving the cause of back pain focuses first on whether the pain is acute (present for less than 6 weeks) or chronic (present for more than 6 weeks). In either case, the scheme-inductive process emphasizes the necessity of assessing for the presence of "red flags;" that is, evidence of any of the nonmechanical causes of lower back pain presented in Fig. 7-9. The red flags in this case are (1) lower back pain at night or rest, (2) unexplained recent weight loss, and (3) recent onset of urination dysfunction.

CASE 4

A 45 year-old woman has made an appointment with her primary care physician to seek treatment for dysphagia (difficulty in swallowing). The following is a transcript of the history taken by the physician and a summary of the physical exam findings:

How are you doing Mrs. Sransky?

- Well, doctor, I'm having trouble swallowing.

What does it feel like when you have trouble swallowing?

- Well, sometimes I'll swallow something and I can feel it stuck down here (the patient points with her right hand to an area just below the sternum of the rib cage) (Fig. 7-12).

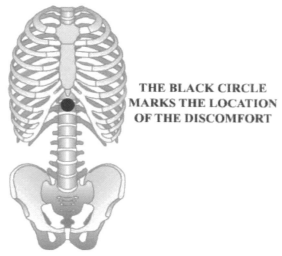

THE BLACK CIRCLE MARKS THE LOCATION OF THE DISCOMFORT

Fig. 7-12: Patient's site of dysphagia discomfort.

Do you have pain when it feels like food is stuck?

- A little bit if I've swallowed something like a bit of an apple or a small piece of meat. But, mainly I just get this uncomfortable feeling that some food is stuck down there.

Do you also have trouble swallowing liquids?

- Generally, yes, in the same place.

When did you notice this problem beginning?

- Oh, it started about two months ago, and it's been getting worse.

What do you mean that it's getting worse; is the pain or discomfort worse or is it happening more frequently?

- Oh, more frequently.

Does any of the food ever come up?

- Oh, yes. That's very unpleasant.

Do you ever have heartburn?

- Well, may be every now and then, but it's not a lot.

Do you have any other problems?

- Well, I've noticed that it's made me loose a few pounds.

Physical Exam Findings: Vital signs are normal. System exams are normal.

Before turning the page, try to write 1 or 2 sentences with semantic qualifiers that succinctly describe the patient's condition.

The following statement is a superior, student team-generated problem representation of the patient: The patient is a 45 year-old female with recent dysphagia of both solid and liquid food that is accompanied by occasional regurgitation and heartburn. There has also been recent weight loss.

As student teams research the pathophysiological mechanism of the patient's condition and discuss their findings in faculty-facilitated class discussion, it is anticipated that the students would achieve the following basic medical and clinical science learning objectives:

1: A student should be able to describe the structure and function of the esophagus in the digestive system.

The esophagus begins in the neck as a continuation of the pharynx; the pharynx is a funnel-shaped muscular tube in the head and neck that opens into the back of the mouth (Fig. 7-13). The esophagus ends in the abdomen at its junction with the cardiac opening of the stomach; the cardiac opening of the stomach is the stomach's upper opening. The junction between the stomach and esophagus is called the gastroesophageal junction. When food is swallowed, it moves within a few seconds from the back of the mouth into the pharynx, down the pharynx into the esophagus, and, finally, down the esophagus into the stomach.

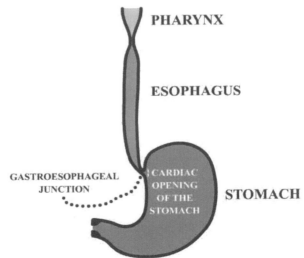

Fig. 7-13: Anterior view of pharynx, esophagus and stomach.

The wall of the esophagus consists mainly of an inner lining surrounded by a major muscle layer called the muscularis externa. Within the muscularis externa there is a nerve plexus called the myenteric plexus (or Auerbach's plexus, in honor of the 19th Century German anatomist Leopold Auerbach who described the plexus). The myenteric plexus is involved in coordinating the peristaltic movements that propel foodstuffs down the esophagus.

Observe in Fig. 7-13 that the esophagus, under resting conditions, is closed off at its upper and lower ends. These sites of closure are called the upper and lower esophageal sphincters. The upper and lower esophageal sphincters are not anatomical sphincters but rather physiological sphincters. In other words, there is no thickening or special organization of muscle fibers at the upper and lower ends of the esophageal muscularis externa to account for the sphincters. Instead, it is the physiological states of the muscle fibers near or at the upper and lower ends of the esophagus that account for the sphincters. The upper esophageal sphincter is largely the result of the resting contraction (that is, the tonic contraction) of skeletal muscle fibers in the lower end of the wall of the pharynx. The lower esophageal sphincter is the result of the resting contraction of smooth muscle fibers of the muscularis externa in the lower end of the wall of the esophagus. Gastroenterologists frequently refer to the Lower Esophageal Sphincter as the LES. The LES is very important because it prevents reflux (that is, backward flow) of stomach contents into the esophagus. The glands in the inner lining of the stomach produce a secretion called gastric juice that is very strongly acidic because of its high concentration of hydrochloric acid. The capacity of the LES to prevent reflux of stomach contents into the esophagus is the main mechanism for protecting the esophageal inner lining from the strong acidity of gastric juice.

2: A student should be able to describe the difference between the two major categories of dysphagia: oropharyngeal dysphagia versus esophageal dysphagia.

Whereas oropharyngeal dysphagia is difficulty initiating swallowing, esophageal dysphagia is difficulty in the passage of food through the esophagus (Fig. 7-14). The physician recognized that the patient was complaining of esophageal dysphagia when she described her problem as a discomfort located immediately below the sternum of the rib cage. The oropharynx is the region of the pharynx that lies immediately posterior to the mouth.

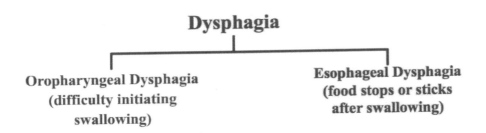

Fig. 7-14: Scheme of major causes of dysphagia.
[Ref: Coderre S, Mandin H, Harasym PH, and GH Fick. Diagnostic Reasoning Strategies and Diagnostic Success. Medical Education (2003) 37:695–703. p. 703.]

3: A student should be able to recall the two major categories of esophageal dysphagia and the semantic qualifiers that differentiate among the specific diagnoses in each major category.

The etiology of esophageal dysphagia can be divided into mechanical obstruction versus neuromuscular disorder (Fig. 7-15). The physician began positing a neuromuscular disorder as the cause of the patient's dysphasia when the patient noted that her dysphagia occurs with both solid and liquid food. If a patient reports dysphagia with solid food only, then mechanical obstruction is indicated.

With respect to diagnostic differentiation among the mechanical obstruction causes, if a patient reports intermittent (occasional) obstruction of solid food only, then a lower esophageal ring is suggested. Esophageal rings are common structural abnormalities in the esophagus. An esophageal ring is literally a concentric ring of esophageal tissue that extends into the esophageal lumen. If a patient reports progressively worsening obstruction of solid food only accompanied by chronic heartburn but no weight loss, then a peptic stricture should be considered. Peptic strictures are strictures of the esophagus that result from diseases either intrinsic or extrinsic to the esophagus. If a patient 50 years of age or older reports weight loss accompanying progressive worsening obstruction of solid food only, then esophageal cancer should be considered. A lifestyle habit of combining cigarette smoking with alcohol consumption increases the likelihood of occurrence of esophageal cancer.

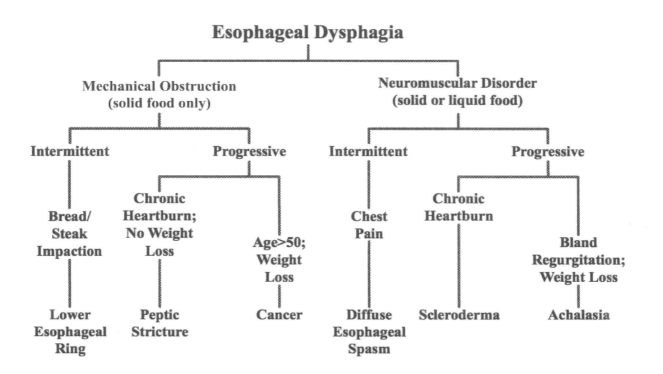

Fig. 7-15: Scheme of esophageal dysphagia.
[Ref: Coderre S, Mandin H, Harasym PH, and GH Fick. Diagnostic Reasoning Strategies and Diagnostic Success. Medical Education (2003) 37:695–703. p. 703.]

In the case under consideration, the patient reports progressively worsening dysphagia accompanied by weight loss and occasional regurgitation and heartburn. Of the three neuromuscular disorders that cause esophageal dysphagia, the clinical picture of achalasia most closely resembles the findings from the patient's history. Although scleroderma is a disease characterized by chronic inflammation of the gastrointestinal tract and other organ systems, it is a less likely diagnosis because it is a disease that also causes indurated (that is, hardened) and thickened skin.

Achalasia is a motor disorder of the esophagus in which the LES fails to relax sufficiently to permit the passage of food morsels into the stomach (the term achalasia is derived from the Greek word that literally means "failure to relax"). This condition typically leads to the retention of food morsels in and dilation of the lower esophagus. Achalasia is associated histologically with a decrease in the number of neurons in the myenteric plexus. The etiology of achalasia is not known.

It is important to observe that although the scheme of esophageal dysphagia in Fig. 7-15 suggests that achalasia in the most likely diagnosis, the scheme does not, by contrast, preclude the possibility of esophageal cancer. In this case, it would be prudent for the physician to order tests that differentiate between achalasia and esophageal cancer.

4: A student should be able to recall an illness script for achalasia similar to the illness script presented here:

ILLNESS SCRIPT
FOR ACHALASIA

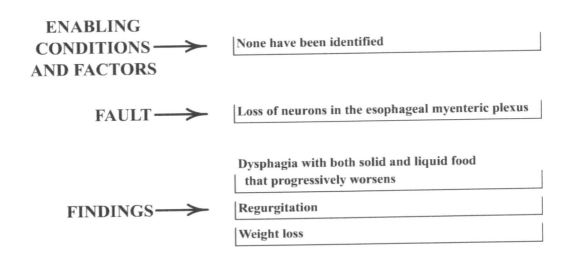

ENABLING
CONDITIONS ——➤ | None have been identified
AND FACTORS

FAULT ——➤ | Loss of neurons in the esophageal myenteric plexus

FINDINGS ——➤ | Dysphagia with both solid and liquid food that progressively worsens
| Regurgitation
| Weight loss

In the clinical presentation curriculum developed by the University of Calgary Faculty of Medicine, a clinical presentation of dysphagia represents a gastrointestinal disorder.

A 57 year-old woman has made an appointment with her primary care physician to seek treatment for pain while walking. The following is a transcript of the history taken by the physician and a summary of the physical exam findings:

How are you Mrs. Krans?
- Oh, doctor, I'm having trouble walking. I like to walk for exercise, but I'm really finding that it's become very difficult for me to do that.

What about your walking is giving you trouble?
- Well, if I walk too long, my right leg starts hurting.

Does your left leg also start hurting?
- No.

Where is the pain in your right leg?
- Below my knee.

Can you recall how long you have had pain in your right leg when walking?
- I'm not sure, maybe for 5 or 6 months. The pain wasn't so bad when I first began to notice it, but ever since then, the pain has been slowly getting worse.

Do you recall if you fell down or suffered an injury shortly before the pain in your right leg started?
- No, nothing like that happened.

Is your right leg ever painful when you are lying down?
- No, not at all.

How about when you're sitting?
- No.

Does bending your back in any way either worsen or relieve your leg pain?
- No.

Does picking up something that's heavy worsen the pain in your right leg?
- No.

Is your right leg ever painful if you're just standing or walking around in your house?

- No, that does not seem to be a problem.

When does the pain in your right leg start when you're walking?

- Oh, I can walk now for only about 2 or 3 blocks before the pain starts. Then, I have to stop and sit down somewhere to rest. It takes a few minutes for the pain to go away. I can then get up and start walking again, but the pain starts all over again after I've gone another 2 or 3 blocks.

Have you been experiencing pain in any other parts of your body?

- No.

Do you have any other health problems?

- No.

Physical Exam Findings: 5 ft, 2 in; 200 lbs. BP: 125/80 mm Hg. P: 75 BPM (beats per minute). System exams are normal except for the findings in the right lower limb of 3+ femoral pulses, 2+ popliteal pulses, 2+ pedal pulses, and an ankle-brachial index (ABI) of 0.7. In the left lower limb, the femoral, popliteal, and pedal pulses are all 3+ and the ABI is 1.0. [3+ pulses are pulses of normal strength. 2+ pulses are palpable but weaker than 3+ pulses.]

Before turning the page, try to write 1 or 2 sentences with semantic qualifiers that succinctly describe the patient's condition.

The following statement is a superior, student team-generated problem representation of the patient: The patient is a 57 year-old female with chronic right lower limb pain that extends distally from the knee upon walking a set distance and resolves upon resting. The right lower limb has 3+ femoral pulses, 2+ popliteal pulses, 2+ pedal pulses, and an ankle-brachial index (ABI) of 0.7.

As student teams research the pathophysiological mechanism of the patient's condition and discuss their findings in faculty-facilitated class discussion, it is anticipated that the students would achieve the following basic medical and clinical science learning objectives:

1. A student should be able to define the following underlined expression:
   The ankle-brachial index (ABI) is the ratio of systolic blood pressure at the ankle to that in the arm.

2. A student should be able to recall the normal range of the ankle-brachial index and explain the clinical significance of its measurement.
   The normal range of the ankle-brachial index is 0.9 to 1.1.

- "The ankle-brachial index test is a quick, noninvasive way to check your risk of peripheral artery disease (PAD). Peripheral artery disease is a condition in which the arteries in your legs or arms are narrowed or blocked. People with peripheral artery disease are at a high risk of heart attack, stroke, poor circulation and leg pain. The ankle-brachial index test compares your blood pressure measured at your ankle with your blood pressure measured at your arm. A low ankle-brachial index number can indicate narrowing or blockage of the arteries in your legs, leading to circulatory problems, heart disease or stroke. The ankle-brachial index test is sometimes recommended as part of a series of three tests, including the carotid ultrasound and abdominal ultrasound, to check for blocked or narrowed arteries." [Ref: http://www.mayoclinic.com/health/ankle-brachial-index/MY00074]

3. A student should be able to describe how major arteries are distributed in the lower limb.

In the lower limb as well as in the upper limb, there are generally arteries that extend across opposite sides of the major joints. In the lower limb, this is the case for the hip, knee, and ankle joints. At each of these three major joints of the lower limb, there is either a large artery or a number of smaller arteries that extend across the anterior, or frontal, side of the joint as well as across the posterior, or back, side of the joint. This distribution of arteries across each major joint ensures collateral (that is, alternate) routes by which blood can flow across the joint. The presence of collateral blood flow across a joint is critically important because, if a limb movement at a joint markedly compresses or bends the arteries that extend across one side of the joint, blood flow through those arteries may become significantly diminished. In such instances, the blood flow through the artery or arteries that extend across the opposite side of the joint acts to ensure that blood flow to parts of the limb distal to the joint is not compromised.

Fig. 7-16 shows an anterior view of the major arteries of the lower limb. The external iliac artery, an artery in the abdomen, is the major source of blood supply to the lower limb. The external iliac artery's name changes to the femoral artery as the artery extends into the front of the thigh (anatomists identify arterial segments according to their location within the body). Near the upper end of the thigh, the femoral artery gives rise to its largest branch, the deep artery of the thigh. Upon giving rise to the deep artery of the thigh, the femoral artery descends through the front of the thigh medial to the shaft of the femur (the term medial signifies that the femoral artery is closer to the midline of the body than the shaft of the femur). At the distal (that is, lower) end of the thigh, the femoral artery enters the posterior, or back, region of the knee, which is called the popliteal fossa. The femoral artery's name changes to popliteal artery upon entering the popliteal fossa. At the distal end of the popliteal fossa, the popliteal artery ends by dividing into two arteries: the anterior and posterior tibial arteries. The anterior and posterior tibial arteries descend through the leg, respectively, via the front and back sides of the leg. The anterior tibial artery's name changes to dorsal pedis upon passing in front of the ankle joint and extending into the foot.

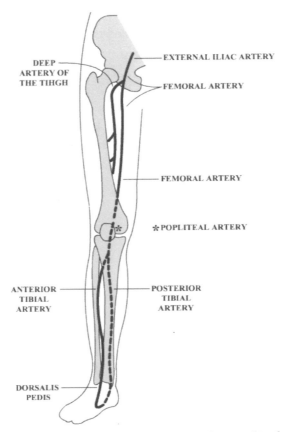

Fig. 7-16: Major arteries of the lower limb.

On the basis of what has been discussed so far, observe that most of the blood supply that extends across the hip joint is conducted across the front of the joint through the femoral artery. There are also smaller arteries that conduct blood across the back of the hip joint; however, they are not displayed in Fig. 7-16. By contrast, most of the blood that extends across the knee joint is conducted across the back of the joint through the popliteal artery. There are also smaller arteries, called genicular arteries, which conduct blood across the front of the knee joint; the genicular arteries are not displayed in Fig. 7-16. Finally, observe that with respect to the ankle joint, the dorsalis pedis conducts blood across the front of the ankle joint, and the posterior tibial artery conducts blood across the back of the ankle joint. In the foot, a branch of the dorsalis pedis, called the deep plantar artery, communicates with the lateral plantar artery branch of the posterior tibial artery.

4: A student should be able to describe the sites in the lower limb at which arterial pulses can be palpated.

There are four sites in the lower limb at which arterial pulses can be palpated:

(1) The femoral artery pulse is palpable in the front of the thigh immediately inferior to the midregion of the inguinal crease.

(2) The popliteal artery pulse is palpable in the back of the knee upon deep palpation of back of the knee with the leg flexed 90° at the knee.

(3) The posterior tibial artery pulse is palpable immediately posteroinferior to (behind and below) the medial malleolus (the medial malleolus is the prominent bony prominence on the medial side of the ankle region).

(4) The dorsalis pedis artery pulse is palpable in front of the ankle immediately lateral to the tendon extending toward the big toe (the tendon of extensor hallucis longus).

5. A student should be able to recall the three major categories of diseases that can produce lower limb pain upon exertion: vascular disease, spinal disease, and lower limb disease (Fig. 7-17).

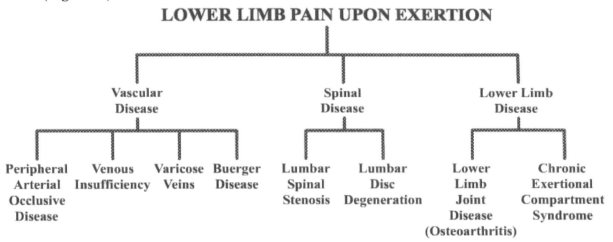

Fig. 7-17: Scheme of lower limb pain upon exertion.

6. A student should be able to explain why an experienced physician would rule out the lower limb diseases as possible causes of the patient's condition.

The physician was able to rule out the lower limb diseases on the basis of the patient's history. Osteoarthritis is not a likely cause because the patient identified her right leg, as opposed to the location of a joint, as the site of her lower limb pain. Chronic exertional compartment syndrome is also not likely as it is a disease most commonly encountered in competitive athletes as a result of very strenuous exercise. The etiology of chronic exertional compartment syndrome is not known. However, like the patient's description of her lower limb pain, the pain of chronic exertional compartment syndrome typically occurs within a defined span of strenuous exercise effort and then tends to subside with rest. The normal daily physical activities that elicit pain in this patient would exclude chronic exertional compartment syndrome.

The term 'compartment' in the name of chronic exertional compartment syndrome refers to the fact that, in the arm, the forearm, the thigh, and the leg, the muscles are all enclosed within tightly wrapped compartments. There are two such muscular compartments in the arm, two in the forearm, three in the thigh, and four in the leg. The muscles in each of these compartments are enveloped within an inelastic, dense sheath of deep fascia [fascia is a term that generally refers to any collection of connective tissue large enough to be described by the unaided eye]. If injury or disease increases the pressure in any of these compartments to the extent that it compromises blood supply to the muscles, there is the risk that necrosis (death) of the entrapped muscles may occur. Chronic exertional compartment syndrome can lead to compartment pressures that compromise blood supply to the muscles.

7. A student should be able to explain why an experienced physician would rule out the spinal diseases as possible causes of the patient's condition.

The physician was able to rule out the spinal diseases on the basis of the patient's history. Lumbar disc degeneration, like herniation of a lumbar disc, can lead to compression of one or more of the spinal nerves that contribute nerve fibers to the nerves of the lower limb and thus lead to radicular pain (that is, pain extending downward to a variable extent within the lower limb). Like lumbar disc herniation, lumbar disc degeneration is a mechanical cause of pain, and thus, as discussed in the case of lower back pain, the pain tends to be affected by activities that involve either spinal movement or pressure changes along the length of the spine. The patient reported that these kinds of activities do not affect her leg pain.

Spinal stenosis is any condition that narrows the spinal canal to the extent that it compresses the spinal cord and the spinal nerves that arise from it (the spinal canal is the passageway in the spine through which the spinal cord extends). Spinal stenosis may occur along any segment of the spine. If the patient's leg pain were the result of spinal stenosis, the stenosis would be in the lumbar region of the spine, as all of her symptoms are confined to the right lower limb. Persons suffering from lumbar spinal stenosis commonly report bilateral, lower limb pain when walking that is relieved by sitting. However, their symptoms differ from the patient in this case in two important respects. First, their lower limb pain is commonly accompanied by numbness or tingling. Second, their lower limb pain typically appears upon just standing from a seated position and then rather quickly is relieved upon sitting down again. The explanation for this second feature of lower limb pain caused by lumbar spinal stenosis is that flexion of the spine, which occurs upon sitting down, relieves the pressure on the spinal cord and spinal nerves in the lumbar region of the spine.

8. A student should be able to describe how veins are distributed in the lower limbs and how lower limb muscles act to pump venous blood from the limbs back toward the heart.

The general distribution of veins in the lower limbs features three categories of veins: (1) superficial veins, (2) deep veins, and (3) perforating, or communicating, veins. The superficial veins extend upward within the superficial fascia of the lower limbs (the superficial fascia is the fascia that lies immediately deep to the skin). The superficial veins receive blood drained from the skin and superficial fascia, and they ultimately empty into deep veins. The deep veins extend upward within the lower limbs; in the thigh and leg, they are aligned parallel to and sandwiched between the bellies of the thigh and leg muscles. The deep veins receive blood drained from muscle and bone tissues. The perforating veins arise from superficial veins, extend into deeper regions of the limbs, and end by joining deep veins.

The superficial, deep, and perforating veins of the lower limbs all have one-way valves. The valves of the superficial veins as well as those of the deep veins are oriented to permit upward but not downward flow of blood. The valves of the perforating veins are oriented to permit blood flow from superficial veins to deep veins but not from deep veins to superficial veins.

Muscle action in the lower limbs contributes significantly to the flow of venous blood from the lower limbs back toward the heart. When thigh and leg muscles contract, the girth of their bellies increase, and the muscles thus squeeze the deep veins between them. This external pressure on the deep veins acts to force open the deep veins' valves and propel blood flow upward through the veins. This action depletes the deep veins of some of their blood. When the thigh and leg muscles subsequently relax and the girth of their bellies diminishes, gravity quickly reverses blood flow in the deep veins. However, the downward flow of blood in the deep veins quickly snaps their valves shut, thus quickly stopping any downward flow. As the blood pressure in the depleted deep veins is now less than that in the superficial and perforating veins, blood flows from the superficial and perforating veins into the deep veins during periods of muscle relaxation. The cycle of muscle contraction and relaxation among thigh and leg muscles thus acts to first directly pump blood flow in deep veins upward and then indirectly pump blood flow from superficial and perforating veins into deep veins.

9. A student should be able to explain why an experienced physician would rule out the venous vascular diseases as possible causes of the patient's condition.

The physician was able to rule out the two venous diseases identified in Fig. 7-17 on the basis of the patient's history and physical exam. The expression venous insufficiency refers to any condition in which there is inadequate drainage of blood from the veins of the lower limbs. Venous insufficiency is most commonly caused by incompetency of the valves in the superficial veins and/or the deep veins of the lower limbs. Varicose veins are veins that have become swollen and exhibit a tortuous path along their length. First, lower limb pain associated with venous insufficiency or varicose veins tends to be alleviated by ambulation (that is, walking) instead of being initiated or aggravated by ambulation. Second, visual examination of the patient's lower limbs did not reveal any varicose superficial veins. However, it should be noted that the absence of varicose superficial veins does not necessarily imply the absence of varicose deep veins.

10. A student should be able to explain why an experienced physician would rule out Buerger disease as a possible cause of the patient's condition.

Of the two arterial diseases identified in Fig. 7-17, the physician was able to rule out Buerger disease, or thromboangiitis obliterans, on the basis of the patient's history. Patients suffering from Buerger disease typically exhibit pain at rest in their hands and/or feet and exhibit cutaneous signs of ischemia in their hands and/or feet.

11. A student should be able to explain how the distribution of lower limb pain in a person suffering from peripheral atherosclerotic occlusive disease serves to identify the site of atherosclerotic occlusion.

Peripheral atherosclerotic occlusive disease (PAOD) is a condition in which medium-sized or larger arteries of the lower limbs become occluded (that is, partially blocked) by atherosclerotic plaques. Atherosclerosis is the pathological process by which cells near the inner lining of an artery accumulate abnormal amounts of lipid droplets to the extent that a flattened lesion called a fatty streak appears. If the pathological process is not abated, the fatty streak is transformed into a relatively large plaque of fibrous tissue that can project into the lumen of the artery to the extent that it interferes with blood flow through the artery. The most common initial symptom of PAOD in a lower limb is muscular pain or fatigue that occurs with ambulation but abates with rest; this symptom is called intermittent claudication, which means intermittent lameness.

Atherosclerotic occlusion of the external iliac artery diminishes blood supply to almost all the lower limb muscles. If the occlusion is significant, the patient thus experiences ambulation-initiated pain extending distally from the buttock.

If significant occlusion of the femoral artery occurs immediately proximal to (that is, before) the origin of the deep artery of the thigh, the patient experiences ambulation-initiated pain extending distally from the thigh. As previously noted, there are three muscle compartments in the thigh; they are called the anterior, medial, and posterior compartments. The femoral artery is the chief source of blood to the anterior thigh muscles, and the deep artery of the thigh is the chief source of blood supply to both the medial and posterior thigh muscles.

If there is significant occlusion of the popliteal artery or the femoral artery distal to (that is, after) the origin of the deep artery of the thigh, the patient experiences ambulation-initiated pain in the leg (anatomists refer to the lower limb region between the knee and ankle joints as the leg). The popliteal artery is the major source of blood supply to muscles in the leg.

Because there is communication between the anterior and posterior tibial arteries in the foot, significant occlusion of either tibial artery does not diminish blood supply to leg muscles, and thus does not produce intermittent claudication.

12: A student should be able to explain why an experienced physician would conclude that peripheral atherosclerotic occlusive disease (PAOD) of either the popliteal artery or the femoral artery distal to the origin of the deep artery of the right thigh is the most likely diagnosis of the patient's condition.

An experienced physician would conclude that PAOD is the most likely diagnosis of the patient's right leg pain because of the following aggregate findings: intermittent claudication, weak popliteal and posterior tibial pulses, and an ABI less than 0.9 in the right lower limb. The combination of no intermittent claudication in the thigh and a femoral pulse of normal strength without any bruits (bruits are abnormal vascular sounds caused by turbulent blood flow) in the patient's right lower limb suggests the absence of any clinically significant atherosclerotic plaques in either the external iliac artery or the femoral artery proximal to the origin of the deep artery of the thigh. The combination of intermittent claudication in the leg, weak popliteal and posterior tibial pulses, and an ABI less than 0.9 all point toward the presence of clinically significant atherosclerotic occlusion of either the popliteal artery or the femoral artery distal to the origin of the deep artery of the right thigh.

13: A student should be able to recall an illness script for peripheral atherosclerotic occlusive disease similar to the illness script presented here:

ILLNESS SCRIPT FOR
PERIPHERAL ATHEROSCLEROTIC OCCLUSIVE DISEASE

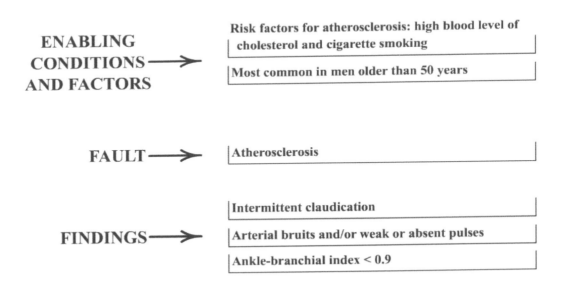

ENABLING CONDITIONS AND FACTORS ⟶
- Risk factors for atherosclerosis: high blood level of cholesterol and cigarette smoking
- Most common in men older than 50 years

FAULT ⟶
- Atherosclerosis

FINDINGS ⟶
- Intermittent claudication
- Arterial bruits and/or weak or absent pulses
- Ankle-branchial index < 0.9

In the clinical presentation curriculum developed by the University of Calgary Faculty of Medicine, the scheme-inductive process for investigating a clinical presentation of pain focuses first on resolving the mechanism of the pain: is the pain the result of (a) disease or injury of some portion of the body's nervous tissues, (b) disease or injury of one of the body's other basic classes of tissues (epithelial, connective, or muscle tissues), or (c) psychogenic in origin? In this case, the finding of weak pulses in the distal part of the painful lower limb quickly identifies the patient's condition as a cardiovascular disorder, namely, peripheral obstructive arterial disease.